Advice to the Young

D1648311

Richard Colgan

Advice to the Young Physician

On the Art of Medicine

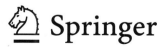 Springer

Richard Colgan
Department of Family &
    Community Medicine
University of Maryland
School of Medicine
29 S. Paca St.
Baltimore MD 21201
USA
rcolgan@som.umaryland.edu

ISBN 978-1-4419-1033-2   e-ISBN 978-1-4419-1034-9
DOI 10.1007/978-1-4419-1034-9
Springer New York Dordrecht Heidelberg London

Library of Congress Control Number: 2009935176

Photo credit: Chemical Hall, Inside view of Davidge Hall, the oldest medical building
still in continuous usage for medical education in the United States, courtesy of Office
of Development, University of Maryland school of Medicine

Printed on acid-free paper

Springer is part of Springer Science+Business Media (www.springer.com)

This book is dedicated to my loving wife Deborah Ann

Acknowledgments

It would be impossible to write a book that involves so many great historical figures without the expertise of others with more knowledge in those respective areas. Foremost, I thank my colleague Milford Foxwell for gifting me with Francis Adam's translation of *The Genuine Works of Hippocrates* and Francis *Peabody's Doctor and Patient*; as well as sharing his excitement of the history of medicine with me. I am equally grateful to another University of Maryland School of Medicine faculty member, Dr. Philip Mackowiak, for his insights and personal recollections of Dr. Theodore Woodward. I would like to acknowledge my mentors, as a student and as a young physician: Dr. Joseph Lombard and Mary Lombard, Drs. David Schneiderman, Michael Berard, and Melvin Sharoky as well as C. Earl Hill. I thank my teachers in private practice: Drs. Michael J. LaPenta, William A. Dabbs, R. Scott Eden, Elizabeth Fronc, and Lisa Murray. I am indebted to my current role models at the University of Maryland School of Medicine, including Vice President for Medical Affairs and Dean E. Albert Reece, our Departmental Chairman David L. Stewart, and the entire faculty of the Department of Family and Community Medicine. I am particularly grateful to the medical students and residents of the University of Maryland School of Medicine who have taught and continue to teach me. One of whom was David Edwards who suggested undertaking this project. I thank Pamela Miller, from the Osler History of Medicine Library at McGill University for her assistance in researching the life of Sir William Osler, and for providing me with archival photos. Lachlan Forrow, President of The Albert Schweitzer Fellowship, was gracious in both assisting me with information about Albert

Schweitzer and allowing me access to photos. My appreciation to Zoe Agoos, from Partners In Health, Boston, MA, for her guidance in helping me learn more about Dr. Paul Farmer and his organization. Gregory Makoul, Chief Academic Officer at Saint Francis Hospital and Medical Center, was kind enough to allow me to include some of his important work on communication skills. I appreciate the counsel and attention to details given to me by Senior Editor Laura Walsh and Editorial Assistant Maureen Tobin from Springer Publishers. Robert B. Taylor and Richard G. Roberts have been extremely generous with their time in providing feedback and offering direction on this manuscript. Imperfections which remain are my responsibility and not theirs. My thanks go to Daniel and Gerard Ricciotti for their expert web designing and videography support. I am especially grateful to the careful review, editing, and suggestions offered by Caitlin Iafolla Zaner-a young healer-whose expertise greatly improved the quality of the book you are about to read.

Lastly but in no way least, I want to acknowledge the most important teachers in my life: John J. and Anna P. Colgan. Together with Eileen Rooney, my wife Deborah, our childern Kathleen, Michael, and Conor, along with my brother John and sisters Jadean, Patricia, and Regina I have learned what love means.

Contents

Chapter 1
Introduction

He knew his art, but not the trade
– Jonathan Swift

Abstract This is a book for the young physician who wants to learn more about the art of medicine. We will explore some of the most important lessons on the ideals of the physician–patient relationship. We will learn about why we do some of the things we do, what our purpose should be, how we can overcome the difficulties sometimes seen in day-to-day doctoring. This book is meant for the idealist who is looking to learn from those before them on how to care for the patient through stories that will both explain and inspire. As one student told me, "Going through medical school, one feels more like a master plumber and electrician of body parts than a healer or a teacher." This book is an effort to help the young physician make the transition from technician to healer by looking at some of the lessons taught by the greatest teachers of medicine through the ages.

John Arbuthnot (1667–1735) served as physician to Queen Anne of England at the turn of the eighteenth century. Recognized by his friends, the English poet Alexander Pope and Anglo-Irish satirist Jonathan Swift, to possess great wit and compassion, John Arbuthnot was not always conscientious about his business affairs; and as a writer he often allowed others to take credit for his work [1]. Swift noted that, as a man, Arbuthnot was "singularly careless of

R. Colgan, *Advice to the Young Physician*,
DOI 10.1007/978-1-4419-1034-9_1,
© Springer Science+Business Media, LLC 2009

his literary fame, published his best things anonymously, and let his friends edit and alter them at will [1]." Upon the death of Queen Anne, Arbuthnot and other members of the queen's court were discharged. Swift lamented this change and said of Arbuthnot's dismissal, "He knew his art but not his trade [1]." Evidently, the distinguished court physician was not an impressive businessman; for this aspect of his profession suffered as he focused solely on the care of his patients. Nevertheless, his nurturing and benevolent characteristics were recognized by his patients and society alike. These values persist to modern day, for it is understood that one of the highest accolades a patient can give his physician is that he or she practices the *art* of medicine.

I have practiced medicine for 25 years and have taught for most of that time. Still, I know that I have not fully mastered the *art* of medicine. However, I think I know something about you, the reader. Each of you knows the importance of mastering the art and is aware of its critical role in delivering total patient care. Yet I suspect you recognize that there is much more to learn. At this point in your training, you view yourself as an incomplete physician. You are idealistic and strive to be a "good doctor," and you truly care about caring for others. Congratulations! This says volumes about you. It means that you know who you are and who you want to be.

You, the reader of this book, are among a self-selected group of high-aspiring physicians and physicians-to-be, joined by numerous other healthcare workers from differing fields, such as nursing, dentistry, pharmacy, social work, clinical psychology, optometry, and podiatry, to name a few. I suspect we all share a common job description. We are a part of the service-to-mankind healing trade. Like those in teaching and law, we are members of the learned professions and of course deserve our distinct recognitions earned through years of hard work and rigorous education. But for the purposes of this book, I am going to simplify matters by referring to the readers as a collective *healer*, since this is the principal group for whom I have written. Similarly, I will refer to the work that we do as medicine, although the subject matter really applies to the wealth of interdisciplinary occupations known as the healing professions.

"I am an incomplete physician. . . who does this guy think he is?" I understand your qualms, for I am an incomplete physician as well. Let me explain: You likely chose medicine as a career for many reasons including a love for science, a respect for mathematics, and an interest in helping others. Maybe you are a natural born surgeon who always loved tinkering, building things, and solving problems. One of the premises of this book is that the best physicians, at least the ones who I would want to be associated with, are lovers of the humanities, of human kind, of *people*. Yet somewhere along the way in your education you have surely noticed a large emphasis on the science—numbers, tests, studies, metrics—and find yourself wanting more of the human side of medicine, the people side. You long to learn more about *the art of medicine*.

I want to tell you how I gained interest in this subject. In between college and medical school, I dabbled in the study of science and considered dedicating my life to this very technical, concrete field. In my interview for a PhD position in Biochemistry at the University of Florida, the chairman said to me, "You look like a people person." I beamed and proudly said, "Yes, I am." He then said, "We are not looking for 'people persons' here. We're looking for someone we can put in a lab; and several months later he'll come out with the answer." I was rejected as an applicant to the University of Florida, only to be accepted into a PhD program in Biochemistry at John Hopkins University. Six months later I left Hopkins, for I was indeed a people person and felt stifled by the confinements of the lab. This book is meant for those who recognize themselves as people persons, for those who see value in the delivery of humanistic health care, and for those who want to hone the skills necessary to practice the art of medicine.

After residency I joined a group of three established physicians, particularly because I wanted to learn from those with greater experience in the practice of medicine. I considered myself well adapted to the intellectual and emotional demands of being a physician, yet I did not appreciate how much I truly had to learn until the respected senior partner told me upon joining the practice, "Don't be discouraged, in about 10 years you'll get in your groove!" Ten years later, I knew he was right. In order to become a better physician, the practice of medicine takes extensive and diligent training, life-long learning, and dedication to the pursuit of evidence-based medicine, as taught by colleagues, students, and patients. After 12 years in private practice, I was given the opportunity to return to academia and pursue a long-standing dream of teaching. Now, as the director of predoctoral education at the University of Maryland School of Medicine's Department of Family and Community Medicine, I am in the position to observe firsthand much of what students and residents are learning.

In order to expose third-year medical students to many of the ideas presented in this book, I developed a workshop in our primary care clerkship that focuses on establishing and nurturing the physician–patient relationship, gaining understanding for the doctor as clinician to the patient and as a gateway to the complex world of health care. I have published research, written scientific articles, reviews, book chapters and provided multiple commentaries on this softer wide of medicine. For many years, I considered assembling these ideas into a book form and was compelled to do so after an MD/PhD student approached me at the end of our clerkship. After expressing similar appreciations he said, "You should write a book Dr. Colgan." He told me that most young researchers are aware of a book by Ramon and Cajal entitled *Advice for a Young Investigator*, and that there is not yet a similar book for physicians or medical students. I was amazed to find this to be the case. I believe strongly that the points made in this book are extremely important for all healers, and therefore I committed myself to taking on this task. To provide a common foundation, I present my personal definition of the art of medicine, which I will largely follow and expand upon throughout this book.

The concept of the *art of medicine* implies much of which is not within the scientific realm. It refers to the interactions between physician and patient, that which falls under the umbrella of humanism. It embodies the stylistic ways in which kindhearted and open-minded physicians practice these traits and signifies the mastery of skill needed for its successful application. Furthermore, this concept entails the more abstract tips, pearls, anecdotes, aphorisms, and best-practiced lessons from exceptional and experienced physicians— those which rarely get disseminated in a formal way to today's young physician or physician-in-training. Understanding the art of medicine raises thought to multiple questions. How it is that someone can meet a physician and within a few moments conclude that he is a good doctor? What happens during an exam room consultation that makes one patient want to follow the physician's advice and another go running for the door? How do we connect with our patients? Why do we want to connect with our patients, and—most importantly—how can we do these things better?

The American educator Francis Weld Peabody communicated the essential quality of a physician is an interest in humanity. Perhaps the single greatest question this book will address is: How can we better show our patients our concern for their humanity? Likewise, how can physicians accomplish this while helping others gain freedom from disease and attain their best possible health? I propose the foundation to this answer is indeed the science of medicine. Knowledge learned from completion of thousands of clinical trials and randomized studies and the intricate scope explored through such technological advancements as electron microscopy and the molecular analysis of the human genome are examples of the *science* of medicine, which has advanced our health. Of course, these must be recognized for their contribution to effective medical practice. My goal is to convey that there is more to medicine than the science, and this notion stems from thousands of years of medical teachings. Even the best practitioners of pure science are incomplete physicians. To be complete physicians, we must appreciate the art of medicine. We must learn how to best use this science for each individual patient and for humankind as a whole, through effective communication, respect, and understanding. Not only this, but we must recognize that the technologies available to restore the health of patients are applied not only to disease processes or organ systems, but to people—with unique backgrounds, cultural values, educations, and life experiences.

"That's fine. I'm with you, so far so good," you might be saying, "So, what's the problem here?" Throughout medical school, residency, specialties, and subspecialties some feel we have allowed the science to overshadow the art. Understandably, the art of medicine is not formally taught to the young physician or physician-in-training. At a minimum, this abstract notion is relegated to passing comments from senior to junior physicians. An example of what such a dialogue might sound like follows:

Junior physician: "How did you get such good judgment?"
Senior physician: "Good experience"
(Long pause)
Junior physician: "How did you gain such good experience?"
Senior physician: "Bad judgment"

This is an example of one of the many ways that junior physicians (medical students, residents, fellows, and those beginning practice) learn the art of medicine—a hall side comment, an informal conversation, the dispensing of a clinical pearl here and there. The main reason why I chose to write this book is because this style of learning—while incredibly valuable—is not universal or consistent, nor are the same critically important lessons taught to each student physician. Some academic medical educators might rightfully argue that such a broad ambition, with a goal of improving outcomes, should not be undertaken unless you have metrics, proven pilot studies, or other data to show that this manner of medical education is "validated." I do not have these things, and I respectfully continue with my goals. Thus, the disclaimer of this book might begin with the fact that this text may not stand up to the rigors of proper pedagogical good form. I acknowledge this, yet I prefer to view the lack of empirical evidence for this form of teaching as testimony to my point that we need to generate a greater discussion of these subjects in medical education. I maintain that we must start somewhere—somehow—to fill in this gap, and I aim to provide what I perceive as some of the most important teachings on the physician–patient relationship as they exist throughout medical history.

Medical schools across the country are evolving to include more on the art of medicine in their curricula. They accomplish this with varying courses described as "Introduction to Clinical Medicine," "The Physician and Patient in Society," "Doctor and Patient," etc. These efforts are excellent, are admirable, and vary from school to school. Extracurricular efforts, as exemplified by the impressive growth of the Gold Humanism Honor Society, for example, and other professionalism efforts are to be lauded as well. They are a start, an important start, but like us they are incomplete.

So why read this book? First, I maintain the belief that each physician wants to be the best they can be. To be a great physician— a true healer—you must be mindful of the tremendous impact which the art of medicine contributes to the entirety of medical practice. Second, it has been my experience that, generally speaking, most physicians are only vaguely familiar with many of the most important lessons from the greatest teachers of medicine. Third, I believe there exists a common recognition among physicians of insufficiency in their education about the art of medicine; moreover, this unfortunate acknowledgement ignites their aspiration for further learning. As I said before, despite nearly three decades of seeing patients and teaching students, residents, and other physicians, I still do not have it right. I am still learning. We have so much to learn from those who came before us. This is what I aspire to teach you. I aim to take you on the best grand rounds on the art of medicine you've ever had.

We will explore what Hippocrates, the Father of Medicine, had to say beyond "*First do no harm.*" We will answer many questions along the way. What did the Greeks and others of Aristotle's time have to teach us about the art of medicine? Why is that you cannot do a rotation in internal medicine without hearing the Canadian medical educator Sir William Osler's name mentioned at least once? Who was he and what was he trying to teach us about being a complete physician? I will introduce you to other greats, such as the previously mentioned American educator Francis Weld Peabody, who had much more to say beyond his most famous quote "The secret in the care of the patient is to care for the patient." We will explore recurring themes which some of the greatest educators spoke of, such as the value of listening to the patient, the demands and rewards of being in the service industry, and why after all is said and done everything we do must come down to taking care of one very important person, our patient.

I recognize that this book is but one physician's viewpoint of the art of medicine, as exemplified by some of the greatest physicians and educators known to mankind. The list is incomplete and qualitative, not quantitative. If in reading this book you are astounded that this person or that person was not included, do not be offended. (And please let me know, so that I might consider them for the revised edition!)

Let me close by repeating my initial reflection—I am not a complete physician. I continuously strive to be a better physician and a better healer by learning from my colleagues, as well as from my patients. I share with you what I believe to be compilations of some of the greatest medical teachers, those who I consider to have exceptional words of wisdom to pass along to all of us. I have much to learn. So do you. But that should not stop us. In the words of English poet and playwright Robert Browning (1812–1889), as he wrote of the poet and scholar Abraham ibn Esra (1092–1167) in the poem *Rabbi Ben Ezra*, I confess to you, "That which I have strived to be, and am not, comforts me [2]." We have an ethical duty to our patients and society to strive for greatness in our personal medical practice. We must attempt to achieve the lessons of French sculptor Rodin who reminds us to "Love your calling with a passion. It is the meaning of your life [3]." Perhaps after reading this book your colleagues and patients will notice a difference in the way you practice medicine, commit to your patient, and strive to connect on a human level in order to provide the best possible care. Above all, my wish for you is that your patients will describe you as someone who "knew the art, but not the trade [1]." Let us begin this journey together.

References

1. Patrick, D. *Chambers Cyclopedia of English Literature*. Philadelphia, PA/London and Edinburgh: J.B. Lippincott Company/W & R Chambers Limited, 1902. 145.
2. Browning, R. *Rabbi Ben Ezra. The Oxford Book of English Mystical Verse*. Eds. Nicholson, D.H.S. and A.H.S. Lee. Oxford: The Clarendon Press, 1917.
3. Rodin, A. Providence Express <http://www.express.org.au/article.aspx?aeid=3246>, accessed May 2009

Further Reading and Resources

Hahn, F.W. *The Art of Medicine*. Kansas City: Leathers Publishing, 2006.

Lacombe, M. *On Being a Doctor*. Philadelphia, PA: American College of Physicians, 1995.

Lown, B. *The Lost Art of Healing: Practicing Compassion in Medicine*. New York: Ballantine Books, 1999.

Lyons, A.S. *Medicine: An Illustrated History*. New York: Harry N. Abrams Inc, 1978.

Ratzan, R.M. and A. Carmichael. *Medicine, A Treasury of Art And Literature*. New York: Harkavy Publishing Service, 1991.

Ramon, S. and Cajal. *Advice for a Young Investigator*. Trans. N. Swanson and L. Swanson Cambridge: MIT Press, 2004.

Reynolds, R. and J. Stone. *On Doctoring*. New York: Simon & Schuster, 2001.

Wear, D. and J. Bickel. *Educating for Professionalism: Creating a Culture of Humanism in Medical Education*. Iowa: University of Iowa Press, 2008

Aspatore Books. *The Art and Science of Being a Doctor: Leading Doctors Reveal the Secrets to Professional and Personal Success As a Doctor*. Boston: Aspatore Books, 2002

Chapter 2
Ancient Times

Abstract Physicians were put on notice in the time of Hammurabi, 1700 years before the common era, that they would be rewarded for a job well done and held personally accountable if in their interactions with their patients harm was done. Not coincidentally perhaps, 1300 years later Hippocrates issued his first rule of medicine: "first do no harm." In ancient times, we saw the physician's understanding of illness move away from a long-held belief that suffering was an expression of God's displeasure, to how illness began to be explained by studying the patient. The skills of observation were highlighted by Hippocrates, with the promise that if the physician was discerning enough, evaluated honestly, assisted nature in prescribing therapeutics he may also prognosticate what would yet be seen. The ancient Greeks laid some of the most important foundations of the art of medicine, as we know it today. Some of the most important tenets of good doctoring and ethical practice can be traced back to Hippocrates, Socrates, and Plato. In this chapter we explore the origin of some important traits which great healers share: temperance, modesty, the power of teaching our patients, and learning from our patients.

2.1 Hammurabi

Freedom from disease is the first blessing
– Siddartha Gotama

R. Colgan, *Advice to the Young Physician*,
DOI 10.1007/978-1-4419-1034-9_2,
© Springer Science+Business Media, LLC 2009

Reverence for good health has been documented since the beginning of recorded history. Siddartha Gotama (563 BCE–483 BCE), the great spiritual leader from India and the founder of Buddhism, inscribed his philosophies on the importance of good health as far back as 500 BCE. Historically, many cultures have allowed the medical practitioner to enjoy a distinguished—even holy—place in society, respected in the same manner as spiritual or religious leaders and philosophers. Medicine is truly one of the greatest vocations a man or woman can devote their life toward. It creates opportunity for individuals to provide service to society as healers, teachers, and respected role models. Many cultures recognize the special and complex part medical practitioners play in directly affecting the health of their people. Physicians are rewarded for a job well done, yet are held responsible when their work is acknowledged or perceived as less than satisfactory. This theme has threaded itself throughout time, with origins as far back as known recorded history.

Societies have held physicians accountable for their conduct since well before the time of 6th Babylonian King Hammurabi (ca. 1795–1750 BCE). The *Code of Hammurabi* represents perhaps one of the earliest of recorded laws, consisting of a total of 282 edicts carved into a 6-foot tall stone monument for all to see. Prominently displayed is the code of patient care, which reads

> If a physician make a large incision with an operating knife and cure it, or if he open a tumor (over the eye) with an operating knife, and saves the eye, he shall receive ten shekels in money. ... If a physician heals the broken bone or diseased soft part of a man, the patient shall pay the physician five shekels in money [1].

This concept rings true to the modern understanding of the physician–patient interaction. A health service is provided and upon completion is compensated. Today there are many expectations about what constitutes a successful interaction, which stem from both objective rules of proper procedure established by decades of scientific research and subjective ideals, values, and thoughts unique to each patient. Completing an "unsuccessful" health encounter certainly has consequences today; however, if you did harm in the era of the Babylonian empire you would suffer an extremely severe punishment. Also included in Hammurabi's rules are the consequences for an unsatisfactory job:

> If a physician makes a large incision with an operating knife, and kills
> him, or opens a tumor with an operating knife, and cuts out the eye, his
> hands shall be cut off. . . [1]

Whether we like it or not, society continues to hold us accountable for all interpretations of unsuccessful care. Of course, avoiding
mutilation or reprimand is not why we want to be excellent healers; however, current thoughts about punishment or consequences
for a physician who has not fulfilled his or her expectations often
echo this sentiment. It is important to remember that we have been
granted special rights by the people whom we serve. We are fidu-
ciaries to a wealth of knowledge, services, and information that will
directly affect our patients' health, and because of this we wield an
incredible power. How do we harness and channel this power toward
the good of our patients?

In this book, we will look at some of the earliest lessons of the art
of medicine, handed down by teachers from as far back as more than
a century ago. We are privileged to make our way down a road that
is well traveled by those who have come before us, those who have
truly learned the intricate and sometimes obscure secrets of patient
care. To begin this story, we must start with the Greeks.

2.2 Hippocrates

> Medicine is of all the Arts the most noble; but, owing to the ignorance of
> those who practice it, and of those who, inconsiderately, form a judgment
> of them, it is at present behind all the arts [2] – Hippocrates (460 BC–?
> 356)

Even 2000 years ago physicians struggled to learn about the *art*
of medicine, and philosophers contributed much to its interpretation. Although he is highly recognized as the Father of Medicine,
little is known about Hippocrates of Cos, also known as Hippocrates
the Great (460 BCE–?356). Two hundred years after his death the
Greeks founded the Library of Alexandria, with the aim to com-
pile and organize thousands of medical writings provided by many
medical, religious, and spiritual philosophers. Works attributed to
Hippocrates stood out for the detailed nature in which the author
described those sufferings from diseases. All writings that seemed to
follow this unique style were thereafter noted as having been written

by Hippocrates and represent the Corpus Hippocraticum—the bodies of work that followed his distinguished theories about health and humanity. Although all of the texts of the Corpus Hippocraticum follow his spoken philosophies and detailed style of analysis, experts agree that many of the works attributed to this collection were certainly not penned by Hippocrates.[1]

Throughout my career, the majority of medical students I have encountered are unable to cite much more about Hippocrates than the famously quoted "Primum non nocere" or "First do no harm." If you had to remember only one line attributed to Hippocrates, this is undoubtedly the most important one to remember, and it is a theme that spans the entirety of medical practice, yet there is so much more that is learned from Hippocrates as one explores his life, personal experiences, and teachings.

Hippocrates was renowned for his power of observation, thought by many to be his greatest skill. In a collection of his writings entitled *Aphorisms* there are over 200 observations of medical practice, disease process, and pathological theory [2]. Many of these are still relevant today, and those that are not as applicable to modern medical practice are of great interest as they provide insight into the evolution of medicine. Furthermore, although some of his conclusions have been shown to be made without current standards of scientific validation, it is important to recognize the value Hippocrates placed on the physician's skill of observation and its application to the patient. This is as important today as it was over two millennia ago. A few of Hippocrates observations from *Aphorisms* follow:

1. Life is short and the art long, the occasion fleeting, experience fallacious, and judgment difficult. The physician must not only be prepared to do what is right himself but also to make the patient, the attendants, and externals cooperate.

---

[1]One of the most frequently cited English translations of Hippocratic texts was written by the Scottish surgeon, Francis Adams in 1849 [2]. The reader is referred to this text to learn more about the veracity of different treatises ascribed to Hippocrates. Suffice it to say that for the remainder of the discussion on Hippocrates I will refer to these writings as being by Hippocrates, with the understanding that it cannot be proven that he actually wrote what has been attributed to him.

2. For extreme diseases, extreme methods of cure, as to restrictions, are most suitable.
3. Spontaneous lassitude indicates disease.
4. Persons who are naturally fat are apt to die earlier than those who are slender.
5. In whatever part of the body heat or cold is seated, there is disease.
6. If erysipelas of the womb seizes a woman with child, it will probably prove fatal.
7. Pneumonia coming on pleurisy is bad.
8. Delirium upon division of the cranium, if it penetrates into the cavity of the head, is bad.
9. When bubbles settle on the surface of urine, they indicate disease of the kidneys and that the complaint will be protracted.
10. Sleep and watchfulness, both of them when immoderate, constitute disease.

Some aphorisms may make you laugh, such as

1. Drinking strong wine cures hunger.
2. If you wish to stop the menses in a woman, apply as large a cupping instrument as possible to the breasts.
3. A woman does not become ambidextrous.
4. Eunuchs do not take the gout nor become bald.

The requirement for careful observation was greatly impressed upon me as a medical student. I clearly remember lessons such as whenever you visit a patient in the hospital you should not leave without paying close attention to the surroundings. It is important to notice even such seemingly plain facts as what objects are on the patient's bedside table, which friends and family members have or have not come to visit them, or the name of the medication label on the intravenous bag. You just might discover something that will help you understand and know your patient better, shed light on unique attitudes and expectations, or just simply enable you to more effectively care for this patient. The skill of observation is one that I emphasize to my current medical students as much as possible.

I once entered the room of an African-American gentleman who was admitted the previous night suffering from chest pain. At his bedside sat a book describing the inequality that exists in health-care delivery to minorities. It reminded me that many members of our society experience healthcare disparities and moreover, that this subject was something my patient thought very important. For me to gain the confidence of this particular patient, I knew that I would need to clearly communicate my plan to provide him with the best health care and to follow through on this expectation as well. Some-times by looking at more than the physical patient you will observe factors which will help you help the patient. This can remind you of something profound: that your patient is a complex individual with a unique cultural, social, and religious background. Or it may be something as simple—but equally as important—as finding out that your patient is not receiving the medication you ordered. Given that a 2006 Institute of Medicine report noted that over 1.5 mil-lion adverse drug events occur in the United States each year due to physicians' oversight is an additional reason to be observant [3]. Yogi Berra once said, "You can observe a lot by just watching." All healers do this; some do it better than others.

Some simple but critical observations you do not want to miss include such details as the pack of cigarettes in your patient's pocket, how your patient just crossed her arms as you gave advice she dis-agrees with and how this may negatively affect her compliance, and the atypical skin lesion which catches your eye as you listen to your patient's posterior thorax. Another subtle observation not to be missed might include the slight change in mental status of an elderly patient, potentially denoting an early sign of sepsis or dementia. When I was a third-year medical student, one professor explained to me, "The organs of the aged do not cry out in pain." I have remembered this throughout my years of clinical practice and it has served me well. Observe all.

Hippocrates cautioned that we evaluate *honestly*. The fact that physicians of his time were observed as being less than honest speaks of the human frailties we are all susceptible to. We have all heard stories or perhaps been witness to physicians today who do not evaluate honestly. The Hippocratic Oath, recited by most medical students prior to graduation, is one way to teach us to act in a profes-sional manner and not provide therapy for our patients, which only serves to bring financial gain. "I will not cut persons laboring under the stone but will leave this to be done by those who are practitioners of this work," Hippocrates wrote in *The Oath* [2]. Many occupations refer to themselves as "professional," but this term takes on a very complex meaning when it is used to denote a physician, dentist, nurse, or other health practitioner. Below is a definition of the professional, as described by a rising third-year student in response to her University of Maryland School of Medicine's application essay prompt:

Entering a profession implies embracing every aspect of a practice through diligence and devotion, that motivates one to develop their skills in an area of academia in order to grow as an individual; moreover, to use this growth as a means to satisfactorily provide a service to their community. A professional is someone who has worked rigorously to learn their craft, and loyally dedicates their time and effort to perfecting it; yet at the same time realizes that perfection is not easily attainable, nor is it guaranteed. Nonetheless, they pursue the goal of professional and self fulfillment through constant intellectual, spiritual and self-actualizing growth. Their profession is constantly progressing and expanding and is interdisciplinary in the knowledge, social, and communicatory skills needed to effectively impact its seekers. Entering into a profession is not a simple proclamation of what one is going to accomplish. Rather, it is an embarkation that wholly encompasses every aspect of that person. It is a declaration of where one's future will take them and, most importantly, the efforts to make this possible through important life choices and significant dedication to those choices. Entering into a profession is an exciting journey, a life changing commitment to service that will better one's community. Not only this, but it is entry into a greater, more expansive domain of professionals. A profession cannot exist through the efforts of just one person, and entering into one must also convey the professional's understanding and embracing of the need to work with others in order to have a successful and respected career. Entering a profession is the first step toward one's fulfilling career in providing a necessary service to society and the greater human good [4].

In the healing arts, the practical and simplified definition of professionalism implies that the professional will follow a course of action that is best for the patient, even at the expense of what may be best financially or personally for him- or herself. The commitment to this notion is symbolically conveyed by recitation of the Hippocratic Oath upon graduation of medical school. Many non-physicians are at least superficially familiar with the Hippocratic Oath, likely because of the great importance it represents not just to physicians but to the public we serve. The Hippocratic Oath follows:

The Hippocratic Oath

I swear by Apollo the physician, and Aesculapius, and Health, and All-heal, and all the gods and goddesses, that, according to my ability and judgment, I will keep this Oath and this stipulation – to reckon him who taught me this Art equally dear to me as my parents, to share my substances with him, and relieve his necessities if required; to look upon his offspring in the same footing as my own brother, and to teach them this art, if they shall wish to learn it, without fee or stipulation; and that by precept, lecture, and every other mode of instruction, I will impart a knowledge of the Arts to my own sons, and those of my teacher, and to disciples bound by a stipulation and oath according to the law of medicine, but to none others. I will follow that system of regimen which, according to my ability and judgment, I consider for the benefit of my patients, and abstain from whatever is deleterious and mischievous. I will give no deadly medicine to any one if asked, nor suggest any such counsel; and in like manner I will not give to a woman a pessary to produce abortion. With purity and holiness I will pass my life and practice my Art. I will not cut persons laboring under the stone, but will not leave this to be done by men who are practitioners of this work. Into whatever house I enter, I will go into them for the benefit of the sick, and will abstain from every voluntary act of mischief and corruption; and further, from the seduction of female or males, or freemen and slaves. Whatever, in connection with my professional practice or not, in connection with it, I see or hear, in the life of men, which ought not to be spoken of abroad, I will not divulge, as reckoning that all such should be kept secret. While I continue to keep this Oath unviolated, may it be granted to me to enjoy life and the practice of the art, respectful by all men, in all times! But should I trespass and violate this Oath, may the reverse be my lot!

The Hippocratic Oath expresses many significant concepts regarding health and healthcare expectations. It is interesting to reflect upon the issues that were felt to be important over two millennia ago and moreover, to recognize that many of these remain controversial in modern times. Clearly these were considered critical and honorable notions at the time of its creation. Have they evolved to mean something different over the centuries? Or are we, as physicians, still learning them?

The idea that physicians should practice beneficently and do what is best for their patients is truly a recurring theme in medicine and society and it will surface many times in this book. This concept is certainly not contentious, but as we will see it is felt by several teachers in the current century to be in need of reiteration. Euthanasia and abortion were clearly concepts, which Hippocrates felt strongly about. Throughout the centuries, these topics evoke strong emotions from both patient and healthcare provider and continue to polarize many people in medicine, politics, religion, and society. It is up to the physician to sort through his or her own values on these controversial subjects and decide their practices accordingly. This is followed in the oath by a declaration that as healers we should live a life of purity and holiness. From this interpretation, it almost sounds like we are entering a religious order, yet the analogy that the healer's examining room is often likened to a confessional strengthens this notion. It may be a stretch to compare practicing physicians to priests; however, in both instances those seeking service divulge the innermost secrets about their bodies and personal lives to a trustworthy advisor. Both physicians and religious figures are healers of people, and like priests, rabbis, and teachers we share a common vocation dedicated to serving society.

Passion follows next in the Hippocratic Oath. While it is important to show compassion for our patients, Hippocrates notes it is not appropriate to be passionate with our patients. Unfortunately throughout the United States and the world of medicine, there continues to be reports of physicians who engage in inappropriate relationships with their patients. It is beyond the scope of this book to discuss in detail what may or may not represent an inappropriate relationship or to impose certain morals or excuse exceptional situations. Suffice it to say that the American Psychiatric Association has decreed that a sexual relationship with any patient, past, present, or future, is not advised. It is important to remember that although both physician and patient are human, protocol and professional expectation creates boundaries that must be followed to provide unbiased and effective care.

Perhaps one of the most important notions emphasized in the oath is that of physician–patient confidentiality. The Hippocratic Oath reminds us that we should not divulge what we have learned from our patients. Our communications and patient interactions must be kept secret in order to maintain patient trust, safety, dignity, and uphold the protocol established by past professionals. In the United States, the recently enacted Health Insurance Privacy and Portability Act (HIPPA) governmental laws serve to emphasize this point. HIPPA was enacted by the United States Congress in 1996. The privacy rule took effect on April 14, 2003, and regulates the use and disclosure of protected health information, including the medical record, by healthcare providers. Someone faithful to the Hippocratic Oath, with goals of maintaining professionalism and upholding the written laws surrounding the consequences of digression, will not divulge any details of one patient's care to another who did not have consent or the express need to know.

The temptation to break this ethic can be subtle and seemingly innocent. An example that I will never forget occurred when one of my patients let me know that her best friend, also one of my patients, was not doing well. She requested that I contact her friend to check in. After what seemed like a minute or two, I did not reply to her. When she asked me specifically what I was going to do about this situation I told her, "I cannot discuss with you whether I do, or do not see Mrs. _____. If she were a patient of mine, I would not be at liberty to speak to another person about her care." The concerned friend under my immediate care became livid in the exam room, raised her voice, and stormed out of the office. She angrily pointed a finger at me as she left and threatened, "If anything happens to her, I will hold you responsible." This situation is a dramatic example, but it illustrates the importance of upholding your standards for all patients, even if they are close friends or family with each other. A much less spectacular example of this is the time I bumped into a patient in the food store. After a friendly greeting, he told me that his boss, also my patient, told him of a recent visit to my office. I think you can guess my reply. It may seem overprotective, but it is important to keep in mind that even the most innocent or seemingly benign invitations to divulge knowledge about another patient must be respectfully declined. This must be done in such a manner that you do not infer that, yes, you did see this patient. To do so without consent would not be professional or legal.

Hippocrates urged that when it comes to therapeutics we should "assist nature." He strongly advocated the encouragement of patients to take better care of themselves by changing their lifestyles, particularly when it came to following a prescribed diet. "A slender and restricted diet is always dangerous in chronic diseases." Likewise, Hippocrates advocated exercise or activity for certain ailments. "It should be kept in mind that exercise strengthens, and inactivity weakens." Although many of his prescriptions would now be viewed as ludicrous by today's standards, his concern for well-being is parallel to current medical practice's mindfulness of the importance of diet, exercise, and activity with regard to patient's health. In recent years, this concept has become more applicable with the overwhelming surge of metabolic syndrome diagnosis, childhood and adult onset diabetes, obesity, coronary artery disease, hypertension, and many other preventable health problems currently plaguing our country.

According to Hippocrates, one of the important qualities for a physician to cultivate is the ability to prognosticate.

> For by foreseeing and foretelling, in the presence of the sick, the present, the past, and the future, and explaining the omissions which patients have been guilty of, he will be the more readily believed to be acquainted with the circumstances of the sick; so that men will have confidence to entrust themselves to such a physician... He will manage the cure best who has foreseen what is to happen from the present state of matters [2].

In the *Book of Prognostics* (c. 400 BC) we also learn one way in which Hippocrates avoided the malpractice of his day—*censure* [2]. This implies that by being aware of the natural history of a disease and whether or not medical intervention will indeed improve a condition, the physician would best be able to counsel a patient about what to expect in the course and outcome of their illness. In the age of Hippocrates, it was recognized that effective communication between physician and patient was one of the best ways to avoid censure, particularly in matters when the prognosis was poor. Honest information about what the patient should or should not expect regarding his or her illness was as important then as it is now. Not only does it base the patient's apprehensions in reality but it also allows for informed decision-making of both parties involved. Furthermore, it strengthens the physician–patient relationship as the patient's trust in his or her doctor is reaffirmed.

In acute diseases the physician should first observe the "countenance" of the patient. Hippocrates compiled some prognostic indications of a poor patient outcome, which are still recognized as valid. These are listed below:

- Hollow eyes.
- Collapsed temple.
- Cold ears.

- A black, green, livid (black and blue; deathly colored), or lead-colored face.
- Seeing the whites of patients' eyes when they are sleeping.
- Cold sweats to the head, face, or neck (these in acute fever prognosticate death).
- A swelling in the hypochondria (the area that is just underneath the anterior rib cage, to the left and right of the epigastrium bilaterally) that is hard or painful.
- All dropsied (disease with drops, or water, edema, e.g., congestive heart failure) arising from acute diseases is bad.
- It is a bad symptom when the head, hands, and feet are cold while the belly and sides are hot.
- Strong and continued headaches with fever, if any of the deadly symptoms be joined to them, are very fatal.

Others of his prognostics are not as applicable to medical practice today and may be placed under the category of just-plain funny, such as

- It is best when wind passes without noise, but it is better that flatulence should pass even thus than it should be retained.

Hippocrates teachings have stood centuries of scrutiny. In this section, we have only briefly reviewed a few of his lessons. Lessons from the Father of Medicine that still are applicable to the young physician of today are many. Some of the most important lessons I think the reader should learn from Hippocrates follow: first do no harm, observe all, evaluate honestly, prognosticate when you can and when it comes to therapeutics, and assist nature. Additionally healers of any era should recognize that we are not in the practice of medicine for money, but to serve our fellowman and that we would be wise to learn from our predecessors in medicine and by carefully studying our patients. Lastly, it is ideal that we should live our life with purity and holiness as we practice our art. Hopefully I have generated an interest in you to read more about the Father of Medicine and the Corpus Hippocraticum. But there are other Greeks we have to discuss!

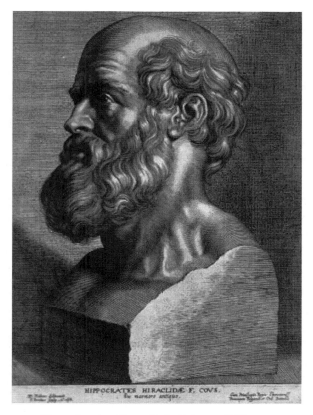

Hippocrates (Engraving by Peter Paul Rubens, 1638, courtesy of the National Library of Medicine, accessed from http://www.encyclopedia.com/topic/Hippocrates.aspx)

2.3 Early Greeks

An incredible part of what we have come to understand as being important to the practice of medicine came from an era when not only Hippocrates but also Aristotle, Socrates, and Plato taught their philosophies.[2] Many students complain about the tortuous and unpleasant experience of being asked esoteric questions, for which the answers are known largely by a more educated senior group. This ritual has even evolved its own derogatory name: "pimping." Interestingly, this style of teaching is similar to the Socratic dialogue, attributed to the classical Greek philosopher Socrates (469 BCE–399 BCE). Put simply, it involves teaching a student by asking questions, such that the student's answers will lead to further questions. This lends itself to understand a greater truth or a more complex lesson.

Much of what is known about Socrates comes from the writings of Plato. From the treatise *The Charmides*, a conversation between Socrates and a young boy, we learn of the importance of temperance. This is a very significant lesson in medicine; in fact, it provides the foundation upon which medicinal practice is built. Medicine is derived from Indo-European *med-*, to take appropriate measures [4]. From the Latin *mederi*, to look after, heal, and cure, stemmed the words medicine and remedy. Other derivates led to the words modern, modest, and moderate. We are urged by Socrates to be temperate, and as healers we can sometimes do the best for our patients by doing the least. As physicians, we become true practitioners of the healing art when we recognize the potential for illness and disease to improve naturally with time and overcome the urge to provide unnecessary physiological therapy. Surgeons in particular are aware of this, the best of whom help their patients by declining an opportunity to operate, in instances when they know it will not benefit the patient.

The word doctor is derived from the Indo-European root *dek-*, to take, to accept, via the Latin *docere*, to teach [5]. It is critical to the physician–patient relationship that we understand the impact and power of our ability to teach our patients. It is too often overlooked. An important lesson for the young healer is to recognize that

---

[2]As with Hippocrates, the mention of these contributors is unfortunately brief and focuses only on illuminating some of the basics of the art of medicine. I hope to expand your horizon and tempt you to want to learn more, to use this text as a springboard for your own literary search.

often it is not "the pill in the hand, but the hand behind the pill" that helps our patients feel better [6]. It is important that we educate our patients about their health so that they may better take care of themselves. A 1998 survey looking at prescription of antimicrobials highlighted this concept. In evaluating attitudes of parents and physicians concerning the prescribing of antimicrobials to a pediatric population, 65% of patients expected to receive an antibiotic for treatment of an upper respiratory infection [7]. In this study there was no correlation between patient satisfaction and receipt of an antibiotic prescription [7]. Instead, patient satisfaction correlated highest with the quality of the physician–patient interaction. Results from focus groups indicate that patients would be satisfied if an antibiotic was not prescribed as long as the physician explained the reasons for the decision to withhold antibiotics [7]. It has also been shown that patients who are informed have lower anxiety and complication rates, compared to those who are uninformed [8–11]. This is *docere* in action!

Another important art we can cultivate in our office visit is to consider asking our patients if there is anything about their illness which they are particularly concerned about. Many patients fear that the symptom they are experiencing may represent something terrible or fatal, which may in fact not be the case at all. Reassurance that in your experience a certain symptom is not at all likely to cause a certain terrible outcome is sometimes the major agenda, which our patients have in making an appointment to see us, even if this concern is not clearly communicated. Other patients focus on what may seem to us as mundane or simple worries, but to the patient addressing these concerns may make all the difference in his or her personal interpretation of the healthcare encounter, its effectiveness, its success, and your abilities as a physician. Being a good prognosticator is truly valued.

During the office visit, it is our responsibility to teach our patients what they can do to take better care of themselves. This may entail specific and clear recommendations about diet, exercise, social habits, such as smoking and drinking or other activities. An excellent way to open the discussion toward teaching your patient is to simply ask them at the end of your visit, "Do you have any questions for me?" We should be clear in giving our opinion as to when they should return in follow up—be it as needed, in 3 months, if condition worsens, etc.—and must strive to set reasonable health goals *with* our patients to emphasize the partnership we are forming to improve their health. Understanding that we are teachers is critical to mastering the healer's art. From the Indo-European root *dek-* of the Latin word *docere* also comes the word *discere*, to learn, from which we get the current derivation disciple [5]. Dignity and decent are also derived from the same Indo-European root. As doctors we are our patients' teachers and must provide them with the environment to learn so as to better their physical and mental wellness. Hippocrates teaches us to be a student of nature, life, and illness by observing all. Others have described this full circle of education by saying "You can't be a good teacher unless you are a good student." We will look further into the importance of being a good student in the next chapter.

References

1. *The Code of Hammurabi.* Trans. L.W. King, 1910. Vol 22, 215–221.
2. *The Genuine Works of Hippocrates.* Trans. F. Adams, 1886. Vol 2, 283.
3. Institute of Medicine, Preventing Medication Errors, Report Brief, Jul 2006 <http://www.iom.edu/File.aspx?ID=35943> accessed May 2009
4. University of Maryland School of Medicine Class of 2011 Admission Essay provided by Caitlin E. Iafolla Zaner.
5. Houghton Mifflin Company, *The American Heritage Dictionary of the English Language,* 4th Ed. Wilmington, DE: Houghton Mifflin Company, 2000.
6. Anonymous
7. Barden, L.S., et. al. "Current attitudes regarding use of antimicrobial agents: results from physician's and parents' focus group discussion." *Clin Pediatr* 1998, 37: 665–671.
8. Cabot, R. "The Use of Truth and Falsehood in Medicine, An Experimental Study," Reprinted in Eds. Reiser, S. et al., *Ethics in Medicine*. Cambridge: MIT Press, 1977. 213–220.
9. Hooker, H.W.. "Truth in Our Intercourse with the Sick," bid., 206–212.
10. Kant, I. "Ethical Duties Towards Others: Truth-fullness," in his *Lectures on Ethics*. New York: Harper Torchbooks, 1963. 224–234.
11. Oken, D. "What to Tell Cancer Patients," Eds. Gorovitz, S. et al., *Moral Problems In Medicine*. Englewood Cliffs, NJ: Prentice-Hall, 1970. 109–115.

Further Reading and Resources

Hammurabi

The Code of Hammurabi. Trans. W. King. 1910. Vol 22, 215–221.

Van De Mieroop, M. *King Hammurabi of Babylon: A Biography*, Oxford: Blackwell Publishing, 2005.

Siddartha

Hesse, H.. *Siddartha*, Los Angeles, CA: Norilana Books, 2007.

Hippocrates

The Genuine Works of Hippocrates, Trans. F. Adams, Baltimore, MD: Williams & Wilkins Co, 1939.

Jacques, J. *Hippocrates: Medicine and Culture*. Trans. M. DeBovoise. Baltimore, MD: The Johns Hopkins University Press, 1998.

Potter, P. *Loeb Classical Library: Hippocrates*. Vol 5. Cambridge, MA: Harvard University Press, 1988.

Lloyd, G. *Hippocratic Writings*. Trans. J. Chadwick. New York: Penguin Classics, 1950.

Early Greeks

Longrigg, J. *Greek Medicine from the Heroic to the Hellenistic Age: A Sourcebook*. London: Duckworth Publishing, 1977.

Sigerist, H. *A History of Medicine, Vol. I and II: Early Greek, Hindu, and Persian Medicine*. Oxford: Oxford University Press, 1961.

Chapter 3
Medieval Medicine

Abstract Three Arabic physicians are highlighted in this section looking at origins of the art of medicine as lived and taught by great physicians in the dark ages. Following a common theme in this book, each physician leader looked back at the collective works and influences of those before them and each was known for advancing more than the art of medicine. Rhazes built on Hippocrates urging of greater usage of the powers of observation to advocating for one of the earliest efforts of scientific inquiry in caring for the patient. Pursuit of the truth in medicine was an important legacy of Rhazes as was his admonition to have humility about the limits of our art. Another Arabic physician, Avicenna was another champion of the power of observation, evidence-based medicine, clinical trials, and the care of the poor. Avicenna recognized that suffering may be due to emotional disorders as well as physical disorders. The third Arabic physician discussed in this chapter was not Islamic as were Rhazes and Avicenna, but a Jewish leader, for whom medicine was a vocation. Moses Maimonides is known by those of the Judaic religion for his theological and philosophical contributions, more so than what he added to the field of medicine. The life he lived and the Oath and Physicians Prayer of Maimonides exemplify the art of medicine.

R. Colgan, *Advice to the Young Physician*,
DOI 10.1007/978-1-4419-1034-9_3,
© Springer Science+Business Media, LLC 2009

3.1 Rhaze

Abu Bakr Muhammad ibn- Zakariya Razi (865 After the Common or Christian Era, ACE – ca. 923 ACE) was one of the greatest physicians of the Middle Ages. Known as Rhazes, this man was regarded as an influential alchemist, philosopher, and Persian scholar. Like so many of the great physicians we will discuss in this book, Rhazes was known not only for what he contributed to the art of medicine, but for his commitment to scholarly work as well.

Historically, Rhazes is remembered for numerous writings on medicine, including pediatrics, ophthalmology, neurosurgery, and pharmacy. A prolific author of his time, he published books and articles in the disciplines of alchemy, religion, and philosophy as well. He is perhaps best known for having authored a nine-volume compendium entitled *Continens Liber* or *The Large Comprehensive*. But the focus of this book is to highlight the contributions which the greatest teachers of medicine have given us as they apply directly to the physician–patient relationship. In short: How is it that we—as medical practitioners—come to regard a specific behavior or style of practice as exemplary medicine? Who can we look to as a role model? Who are the icons that have shown themselves as masters of the art of medicine, specifically as it pertains to the physician–patient relationship? How do we know a medical great when we see one? Rhazes helped us to understand by example what we now recognize as superb practice.

Rhazes advocated for use of the power of observation, and in doing so he encouraged scientific inquiry in caring for the patient. Since the time of Hippocrates, the humoral theory was held by physicians as the basis for their understanding of disease. According to Galen of Pergamum, a prominent philosopher of Greek origin, a person was sick if one of their four humors—black bile, yellow bile, phlegm, and blood—were out of balance. Humoralism was closely linked to the Greeks' theory of four elements—earth, wind, fire, and water. By observing his patients in a specific and particular manner, Rhazes challenged the notions of those before him. He was the first to refute the opinions of Galen in *Doubts About Galen*, which ultimately led to the dismissal of humoralism and its consideration of being non-scientific. This change in thinking did not occur quickly, and Rhazes was met with much resistance for many years. In fact, his thinking was not fully accepted until Rudolph Virchow developed his thesis on cellular pathology in the mid eighteen hundreds.

Rhazes urged practitioners to think independently, to learn from their experiences with disease through meticulous observation and constant questioning. Using these practices himself, he published some of the first scientific descriptions of medical illnesses, and he is even credited with providing the first accounts of such diseases as smallpox and measles. Rhazes also disagreed with Galen over the nature of fever and urinary ailments, basing his opinions on his own practice and patient observations. He taught, "All that is written in books is worth much less than the experience of a wise doctor." Living by his own lessons led him to many discoveries. He was the first to describe allergic rhinitis and asthma in a scientific manner. His writing *A Dissertation on the Cause of the Coryza (acute inflammation of the mucous membranes of the nasal cavities) which Occurs in the Spring When the Roses Give Forth Their Scent* is the first known publication on hay fever.

Rhazes advocated for the practice of evidence-based medicine in the Middle Ages. He developed standards of question and practice that provided the foundation for modern thought on evidence-based medicine, which few physicians would argue against today. Rhazes taught that physicians should look at whether or not a disease was truly curable versus non-curable with implication of multiple treatments; further, they should use the information gained to change their practices for the betterment of the patient. When it came to caring for those with cancer and leprosy, Rhazes urged that the physician not be blamed for his patient's poor outcome. He was a fierce independent thinker who, while urging diligent study and the pursuit of knowledge, also taught humility and caution when it comes to unrealistic expectations of being confident in what we seemingly know. He taught that "truth in medicine is an unattainable goal, and the art as described in books is far beneath the knowledge of an experienced and thoughtful physician [1]."

In addition to promoting the skills of observation and independent thinking, Rhazes argued that we should be ethical and moral about our daily routine:

> "The doctor's aim is to do good, even to our enemies, so much more to our friends, and my profession forbids us to do harm to our kindred, as it is instituted for the benefit and welfare of the human race, and God imposed on physicians the oath not to compose mortiferous remedies [1]."

Although he was a physician to the rich and powerful, Rhazes' devotion to medical education and treatment of the poor made him highly sought after as a teacher by medical students of his day. Rhazes was known for treating the impoverished sick free of charge during a time when medical care by physicians of such repute was mainly enjoyed by those of wealth. He pioneered the teaching of medicine by the bedside, and wrote a self-help, home remedy guide for the common man—recognizing that many could not afford to seek professional medical care.

Rhazes possessed the wise and insightful thinking that physicians should be mindful of their patient's mental health just as well as their physical health. He wrote of the importance of a sound mind and a sound body and discussed the significant positive impact afforded to those physicians humble enough to be friendly with their patients. He has been called "probably the greatest and most original of all Muslim physicians [2]." Rhazes was known as much for his intelligence as for his kindness and compassion to others. He was troubled by poverty and suffering and gave away his fortune, such that he died in destitution.

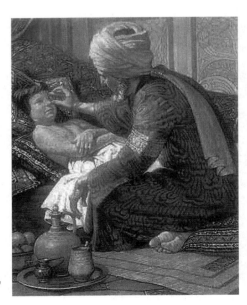

Rhazes (Pictured at the bedside of a young patient afflicted with measles. Accessed from dodd. cmcvellore.ac.in/hom/09% 20-%20Rhazes.jpg)

3.2 Avicenna

Another Arabic teacher of medicine was the Persian physician and philosopher Abu Ali Sinna (980 ACE – 1037 ACE). Also known as Hakim Ibn Sina, he is more commonly known in the west as Avicenna. Avicenna is known as the father of early modern medicine. Like many of the great teachers we discuss in this book, he is known by those outside of medicine for many significant accomplishments. And like other medical giants he was a prolific writer, with hundreds of treatises still in existence. Avicenna's best-known works are *The Book of Healing* and the fourteen-volume *Qanun* or *Canon of Medicine*. Completed in 1025 ACE, it served as a foundation for medical teaching for over 700 years. *The Canon of Medicine* is considered by many to represent the first pharmacopeia, including more than 600 medicinals, chemicals, and physical properties and details of their implementation. Avicenna also wrote of the necessity of studying drugs before exposing them to the public, antedating our current practice of clinical trials by hundreds of years. Avicenna was recognized by Osler as "author of the most famous medical textbook ever written [3]." He noted that Avicenna's *Canon* remained "a medical bible for a longer time than any other work [3]." Copies of an English translation can still be purchased and are the basis for modern-day primary medical pharmaceutical texts.

Like Rhazes, Avicenna is known for promoting the power of observation and experimentation. He practiced evidence-based medicine and helped elucidate the contagious nature of infectious disease, introducing the concept of quarantine to control outbreaks of infections. He cared for the sick—often at no cost—brought to him in great numbers because of his renowned reputation. Avicenna's contribution to the art of medicine may be that he was a thinker, scholar, and someone adept in the intellectual pursuit of diverse topics that affect mankind. In addition, he incorporated thoughts and ideas from those who preceded him, which helped shape his own growth in many disciplines. Avicenna was influenced by Hippocrates, Galen, Aristotle, Rhazes, and many lessons from Indian medicine. This becomes a recurring theme of the great healers, who look to the teachings of others before them for guidance and knowledge in how they should proceed in the practice of their art. You are in good company.

Avicenna incorporated physical, emotional, and spiritual medicine into his system of healing. Like Rhazes, Avicenna also recognized that emotional illness could be expressed in physical complaints. In the *Canon* he describes an illness afflicting a Prince, which puzzled the local doctors for its severity but apparent lack of physical cause. Avicenna noted a fluttering in the Prince's pulse whenever the name or address of his love interest, from whom he was separated, was mentioned. The patient was promptly cured upon being reunited with his lover. Avicenna, like many of the great physicians discussed in this book, was able to recognize that patients complaining of physical symptoms can have an underlying emotional discord as the cause for their discomfort. The ability to rule out organicity and diagnose a patient with a functional disorder is a hallmark of a great healer. This ancient doctor of doctors was a champion for the use of herbals and dietary changes to promote wellness. Like Hippocrates (and many of our mothers), he believed that food was the best medicine. Most of us can surely relate to the admonitions of "Doctor Mom" who extols the virtues of chicken soup, carrots, spinach, and other foods as being good for us.

Avicenna was able to incorporate what he had learned from others and thereby developed a way of caring for his patients in a manner that was best suited for each individual. He promoted scientific study and careful detailing of the medical and pharmaceutical procedures he used on his patients. Further, he used these principles for those who could and could not afford his services and donated his time and efforts to help underserved and impoverished populations. For those he could not directly care for, he offered assistance by developing manuals of health care for the layperson. This is how Avicenna continues to teach us today. He reminds us to look back to our ancestors and learn from them to create new knowledge in a scientific manner and to use the information gained to reach out and heal our current patients.

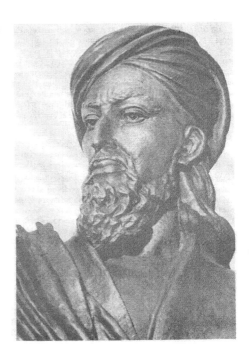

Ibn Sina or Avicenna
(public domain)

3.3 Maimonides

Moses Maimonides (1135 ACE–1204 ACE), also known as Rabbi
Moses ben Maimon or Rambam was perhaps the most famous
Jewish physician in Arabic medicine. Born in Cordova, he later
migrated to Palestine and then to Cairo to avoid religious persecution. This rabbi, Jewish philosopher, scholar, and writer is revered
by those of the Judaic faith, not because of his stature as physician,
but as one of their greatest theologians. As one of my medical students, who is an observant Jew told me, "When we think of Maimonides, his role as a physician is about eighth down on the list for
which he is known for in Judaism." Maimonides wrote a number
of texts, including *Fusul Musa* or *Chapter of Moses*, a collection
of medical aphorisms. When researching the long list of those who
should be considered in a text about the art of medicine as taught by

the masters of medical education, Maimonides name is immediately thrust to the top of this list because of his devotion to his patients and his passion for service.

Maimonides was the physician to a Sultan, and in a letter sent to Samuel (Shmuel) ibn Tibbon he described the typical scene that awaited him at home after a long and brutal day of work:

> "I would find the antechambers filled with people, both Jews and Gentiles, nobles and common people, judges and bailiffs, friends and foes - a mixed multitude, who await the time of my return. I dismount from my animal, wash my hands, go forth to my patients, and entreat them to bear with me while I partake of some slight refreshment, the only meal I take in the twenty-four hours. Then I attend to my patients, write prescriptions and directions for their various ailments. Patients go in and out until nightfall, and sometimes even, I solemnly assure you, until two hours and more in the night. I converse with and prescribe for them while lying down from sheer fatigue, and when night falls I am so exhausted that I can scarcely speak.... I have here related to you only a part of what you would see if you were to visit me [4]."

With regard to the physician–patient relationship, Maimonides' true greatness manifested as a complete commitment to his patients. One can picture this weary man stumbling into his home only to find, amidst the hanging lanterns and dim light, mothers holding their sick children with looks of fear on their faces. Interestingly, Maimonides refers to his practice as *healing*. If you will remember, so did Hammurabi. Maimonides revered the great teachers of medicine who preceded him and singled out Hippocrates as "Head of Physicians." Like Hippocrates, Maimonides taught students of medicine, and advocated that "a physician should begin with simple treatment, trying to cure by hygiene and diet before he administers drugs." Recognizing the lessons of those who come before us is characteristic of many of the physician-teachers highlighted in this book. As Maimonides looked back to Hippocrates for inspiration, so too did Osler look back to Maimonides for his wisdom and highly regarded the Jewish scholar as the "Prince of Physicians."

Maimonides possessed love for his profession, a true dedication to his practice and his patient. He recognized his skill as a gift from God and passionately wrote of this realization. He is thought by some to have expressed these thoughts in *The Physician's Oath and Prayer*. Although the authenticity of this text being penned by Maimonides has been called into serious questioning—felt by others to be the work of Markus Herz (1747–1803), a German physician and pupil of Immanual Kant—this does not detract from the beauty of what follows:

The Physician's Oath and Prayer of Maimonides

The Oath of Maimonides

The eternal providence has appointed me to watch over the life and health of Thy creatures. May the love for my art actuate me at all times; may neither avarice nor miserliness, nor thirst for glory or for a great reputation engage my mind; for the enemies of truth and philanthropy could easily deceive me and make me forgetful of my lofty aim of doing good to Thy children.

May I never see in the patient anything but a fellow creature in pain. Grant me the strength, time and opportunity always to correct what I have acquired, always to extend its domain; for knowledge is immense and the spirit of man can extend indefinitely to enrich itself daily with new requirements.

Today he can discover his errors of yesterday and tomorrow he can obtain a new light on what he thinks himself sure of today. Oh, God, Thou has appointed me to watch over the life and death of Thy creatures; here am I ready for my vocation and now I turn unto my calling [5].

The Prayer of Maimonides

"Almighty God, Thou has created the human body with infinite wisdom. Ten thousand times ten thousand organs hast Thou combined in it that act unceasingly and harmoniously to preserve the whole in all its beauty the body which is the envelope of the immortal soul. They are ever acting in perfect order, agreement and accord. Yet, when the frailty of matter or the unbridling of passions deranges this order or interrupts this accord, then forces clash and the body crumbles into the primal dust from which it came. Thou sendest to man diseases as beneficent messengers to foretell approaching danger and to urge him to avert it.

Thou has blest Thine earth, Thy rivers and Thy mountains with healing substances; they enable Thy creatures to alleviate their sufferings and to heal their illnesses. Thou hast endowed man with the wisdom to relieve the suffering of his brother, to recognize his disorders, to extract the healing substances, to discover their powers and to prepare and to apply them to suit every ill. In Thine Eternal Providence Thou hast chosen me to watch over the life and health of Thy creatures. I am now about to apply myself to the duties of my profession. Support me, Almighty God, in these great labors that they may benefit mankind, for without Thy help not even the least thing will succeed.

Inspire me with love for my art and for Thy creatures. Do not allow thirst for profit, ambition for renown and admiration, to interfere with my profession, for these are the enemies of truth and of love for mankind and they can lead astray in the great task of attending to the welfare of Thy creatures. Preserve the strength of my body and of my soul that they ever be ready to cheerfully help and support rich and poor, good and bad, enemy as well as friend. In the sufferer let me see only the human being. Illumine my mind that it recognize what presents itself and that it may comprehend what is absent or hidden. Let it not fail to see what is visible, but do not permit it to arrogate to itself the power to see what cannot be seen, for delicate and indefinite are the bounds of the great art of caring for the lives and health of Thy creatures. Let me never be absentminded. May no strange thoughts divert my attention at the bedside of the sick, or disturb my mind in its silent labors, for great and sacred are the thoughtful deliberations required to preserve the lives and health of Thy creatures.

Grant that my patients have confidence in me and my art and follow my directions and my counsel. Remove from their midst all charlatans and the whole host of officious relatives and know-all nurses, cruel people who arrogantly frustrate the wisest purposes of our art and often lead Thy creatures to their death.

Should those who are wiser than I wish to improve and instruct me, let my soul gratefully follow their guidance; for vast is the extent of our art. Should conceited fools, however, censure me, then let love for my profession steel me against them, so that I remain steadfast without regard for age, for reputation, or for honor, because surrender would bring to Thy creatures sickness and death.

Imbue my soul with gentleness and calmness when older colleagues, proud of their age, wish to displace me or to scorn me or disdainfully to teach me. May even this be of advantage to me, for they know many things of which I am ignorant, but let not their arrogance give me pain. For they are old and old age is not master of the passions. I also hope to attain old age upon this earth, before Thee, Almighty God!

Let me be contented in everything except in the great science of my profession. Never allow the thought to arise in me that I have attained to sufficient knowledge, but vouchsafe to me the strength, the leisure and the ambition ever to extend my knowledge. For art is great, but the mind of man is ever expanding.

Almighty God! Thou hast chosen me in Thy mercy to watch over the life and death of Thy creatures. I now apply myself to my profession. Support me in this great task so that it may benefit mankind, for without Thy help not even the least thing will succeed."

In the Oath of Maimonides he cites, "Here am I ready for my vocation and now I turn unto my calling." This is one of the earliest times in recorded history that we see the field of medicine being referred to as a vocation and a calling. It is clear that Maimonides viewed his work as a physician as sacred, given to him by God so that he could help his fellow man. Indeed Maimonides states, "Providence Thou hast chosen me to watch over the life and health of Thy creatures." What inspirational words! I do not imagine there is a single reader who feels differently about his *art*. Wouldn't you love to have Maimonides as your doctor? History has noted the greatness of Maimonides for his contributions to religion and philosophy, more so than his contributions to medicine. His service to his people, patients, and students is undeniable in many disciplines. That he inspired others to think led to the Jewish adage of him, attributed to the German-Jewish Philosopher Moses Mendelssohn (1729–1786): "From Moses unto Moses there arose not one like Moses [6]." We are truly fortunate that a healer as devoted and humanistic as Maimonides found an intellectual and spiritual outlet in medicine.

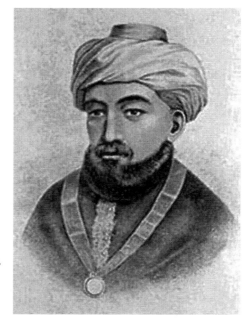

Moses Maimonides (Portrait, 19th century, author unknown. Commonly used image indicating one artist's conception of Maimonides's appearance, accessed from http://commons.wikimedia.org/wiki/File: Maimonides-2.jpg)

References

1. "Islamic Science, the Scholar and Ethics." *FCTC Limited* 24 Feb 2006. 1 May 2009. <http://www.muslimheritage.com/topics/default.cfm? ArticleID=570>
2. Browne, E.G. *Islamic Medicine*. Dehli: Goodword Books Pvt. Ltd., 2001.
3. Osler, W. *The Evolution of Modern Science*. New Haven, CT: Yale University Press, 1921. 243.
4. Illievitz, A.B. "Maimonides The Physician, Responsa Pe'er HaDor." *Can Med Assoc J* Apr 1935. 440–442.
5. *Bull Johns Hopkins Hosp.* Trans. Harry Friedenwald. 1917, 28: 260–261.
6. Chapters on Jewish Literature, Israel Abrahams, Chapter XIII. Moses Maimonides. May 2009. <http://www.authorama.com/chapters-on-jewish-literature-13.html>

Further Reading and Resources

Rhazes

Stolyarov, H., II "Rhazes: The Thinking Western Physician." *The Rational Argumentator* 2002, Issue VI.

Ranking, G.S.A. The Life and Works of Rhazes. In *Proceedings of the Seventeenth International Congress of Medicine*. London, 1913. 237–268.

Avicenna

"Educating Health Professionals: The Avicenna Project." *Lancet* 2008, 371; 9617: 966–967.

Goodman, L.E. *Avicenna*, London: Taylor and Francis, 2003.

Browne, E. *Islamic Medicine*. Dehli: Goodword Publishing, 2002.

Maimonides

Kraemer, J. *Maimonides: The Life and World of One of Civilizations Greatest Minds*. New York: Doubleday, 2008.

"Maimonides, a biography." The Maimonides Heritage Foundation 2005. 20 Feb 2009. <http://www.maimonidesheritage.org/History.asp>

Chapter 4
The Twentieth Century

Abstract The art of medicine had many proponents in the twentieth century. Three of the most significant teachers are discussed in this chapter. Sir William Osler took the art and teaching of medicine to a new level. He urged physicians to use all of their senses when evaluating patients and to show equanimity and imperturbability when practicing medicine. Osler appreciated that an understanding of the psychosomatic basis of illness was important, and he has been referred to as both the father of internal medicine and psychosomatic medicine. Francis Weld Peabody recognized that with the advancement of scientific discoveries care of the patient was sometimes overlooked. He taught that an interest in humanity was an essential quality of a physician. Both Peabody and Osler recognized students in their earliest clinical years as having an excellent opportunity to learn medicine by the bedside. Albert Schweitzer taught the art of medicine by example, having committed to his life to service. His philosophy of reverence for life was also an argument that he lived his life by, in serving the poor at his jungle hospital in Gabon. Schweitzer taught that there was no greater motto one could follow than to live a life of service.

4.1 Sir William Osler

"To each one of you the practice of medicine will be very much as you make it... to one a worry, a care, a perpetual annoyance, to another, a

R. Colgan, *Advice to the Young Physician*,
DOI 10.1007/978-1-4419-1034-9_4,   41

daily joy and a life of as much happiness and usefulness as can well fall
to the lot of man."

– Sir William Osler

One of the most influential English-speaking physicians in history was the Canadian medical educator Sir William Osler (1849–1919). Following postgraduate training in England and Europe, he taught medicine and pathology at many institutions including McGill and the University of Pennsylvania and even became the first professor of medicine at Johns Hopkins University in 1889. In 1905 Osler became Regius Professor of Medicine at Oxford. Sir William Osler's impact on medical education is likely far greater than any other teacher in the history of Western medicine.

Osler is considered the *father* of internal medicine and authored the textbook *The Principles and Practice of Medicine* in 1892, which was widely used for decades. This text inspired John D. Rockefeller to establish the Rockefeller Institute for Medical Research. Osler's description of infectious endocarditis led to his name being associated with infectious nodules—painful, purple, and on the palm—and the soles of afflicted patients (Osler's nodes). But Osler's greatest legacy was as a medical educator. He pioneered the concept of teaching students by having them learn directly from patients. At a time in history when students were largely taught only in classrooms, he championed the concept of gathering knowledge at the bedside. Osler wrote, "He who studies medicine without books sails an uncharted sea, but he who studies medicine without patients does not go to sea at all" [1].

Osler prided himself in his role as a medical professor. He was once quoted, "On my epitaph I would like nothing else written other than. . . 'he taught medical students in the wards,' for I view this by far as the single greatest thing I have ever done" [2]. It is clear that Osler contributed greatly to the science of medicine, lending more documented detail on physiology and disease process than perhaps anyone before him. So what did he have to offer with regards to the art of medicine? Osler indoctrinated two cardinal concepts to his students, that every physician should have (1) *imperturbability* and (2) *aequanimaty*:

Imperturbability means coolness and presence of mind under all circumstances, calmness amid storm, clearness of judgment in moments of grave peril, immobility, passiveness... and the physician who has the misfortune to be without, who betrays indecision and worry, and who shows that he is flustered and flurried in ordinary circumstances, loses rapidly the confidence of patients [1].

Imperturbability comes from wide experience and a deep understanding of the subject matter. Of this notion Osler wrote, "No quality takes higher rank" [1]. He recognized education, practice, and experience would help the student to develop this skill.

I remember a classic example of a young physician, only a year out of medical school, who did *not* showcase his imperturbability in a time of crisis. As a medical student, I observed this new physician called onto the wards to attend to a patient suffering from shock. The patient was with altered mental status, hypotension, and near cardiac arrest. The intern, who to his defense had no desire whatsoever to be a somatic physician, rushed out of the room chaotically. Obviously flustered, waving his arms frantically he shouted to the nurse, "Someone call a doctor!" To which the grounded nurse replied, "You are a doctor!" Ultimately a "code blue" was called and the patient was transferred to the coronary care unit. I am certain that to this day the intern, now a practicing psychiatrist, is thankful that he is far away from the medical wards. The notion of imperturbability is also described in the aphorism "the first pulse you should take in a code is your own." In other words, when faced with an emergency, check yourself to be sure that you are not overreacting or flustered, before looking to render aid. This is easier said than done, particularly for young healers. But do not despair over being of a young age. Osler also felt that "the real work of life is done before the 40th year and that after the 60th year it would be best for the world and best for themselves if men rested from their labours" [3].

According to Osler, an important accompaniment to imperturbability is aequanimaty, defined as the mental embodiment of imperturbability. An example cited in a collection of Osler's works, entitled *Aequanimatus* is the physician's ability to bear, with composure, the misfortune of others. For some this may come as a natural skill. For others, it must be learned. Being patient with those who may not have attained your level of knowledge or experience is a display of aequanimaty. Inherent in this concept is the fact that absolute truth is unattainable and that we must be content in our knowledge that in so many situations in medicine—and in life—we do not hold all the pieces of the puzzle.

This brings me to a critical concept for the young healer. All physicians learn clinical medicine in the wards and in outpatient clerkships. Some students prefer to gather knowledge about clinical medical practice and procedure from readings and lectures. This is essential. Yet most experienced clinicians will tell you that their greatest lessons were taught by preceptors in a clinical setting, as both student and teacher partnered together in caring for a patient. This mentoring is critical in the maturation process of the future physician and provides valuable insight on interactions between different levels of authority, responsibility, and experience in the delivery of health care. Unfortunately, I have never met a medical student who (when asked) did not admit to having been derided or mocked on occasion during this process. The following account of my first clinical rotation in medical school illustrates this point well:

> I was excited to be a third year student in the Emergency Department of a large county hospital after my basic science curriculum, during which I had little clinical exposure. Amid one memorable shift, I was in the process of learning how to change a Foley catheter when the senior resident interrupted my tutorial and yelled aloud to the other staff, "He has no pulse.... CODE BLUE!" To my shock the patient was quickly wheeled from underneath my arms to the cardiac arrest area of the Emergency Room. The ER attending, Dr. Melvin Sharoky, with aequanimaty and imperturbability called for more information about the patient. I tried to speak, but no words escaped until seemingly minutes later when I blurted out, "Schneiderman and Berard." The intern David Schneiderman and medical resident Michael Berard were quickly summoned and assisted as the attending ("one who attends") ran the code. I stood there helplessly, intensely watching the passing of a human life. Then the code was over. Dr. Sharoky said, "I'm calling it," and our patient was pronounced dead.
>
> As is the custom after a cardiac arrest, physicians will pause and discuss the case to try to learn from it—to figure out if something could have been done differently. When asked "What do you think killed the patient?" the ER attending replied. "I'll tell you what I think killed the patient," he said, "I think the medical student killed him by pulling on the Foley catheter." I was stunned. It was my first real memory of being involved in the care of a patient, and I'd heard from the senior physician that I killed a man.

But he was not serious. This was a teaching point, not a true indictment. The lesson was that manipulation of a catheter in a gravely ill man—albeit often necessary—has the potential to induce a vagal response, i.e., the patient's heart rate can decrease, which may be the touché that forces life to leave a man's body. I later learned that our patient died of pneumococcal sepsis and meningitis, a deadly disease, which few escape. But this wise ER attending's teaching point will never leave me: be careful. Another lesson might have been that junior clinicians must get used to taking feedback from their superiors, so as to learn how to practice great medicine. In this setting, as a third year student, I didn't know any better and thought that these comments were meant as a true measure of inadequacy of my involvement in this case. I now know it was not, and that we must accept all types of criticism, lessons, and even sarcasm delivered so as to learn how to care for our patients.

The aforementioned scenario was an example of clinical medical education delivered with good intentions. Learning clinical pearls in academia is not always wrapped in niceties. Sometimes students rightfully perceive that a lesson is being taught in less than a good spirited manner. To the young healer I urge you to not let a colleague or senior teacher put you down or make you feel small for not knowing something. You have either witnessed or seen it happen, I am sure. For example, a student is asked, "What are the five most common types of lymphoma?" to which he replies in exasperation "I don't know... I only know two: Hodgkins and Non-Hodgkins!" This is followed by the smug teacher slowly walking away with a smirk and a sense of false victory. Pity these educators for they do not have the knowledge to know that they make themselves inferior, not superior, by attempting to put you down. In fact, I believe that one of the smartest answers to any question is, "I don't know... but I will look it up and get back to you." Pity any hubristic colleague who might attempt to disrespect you in such a way and then teach them.

Osler made many contributions to clinical medicine, including helping to create the system of residency training that is still used today. But again, I must remind myself and the reader that, rather than a proper history of medicine text, in this book we look to learn from the greatest teachers of medicine for what they taught about the *art* of medicine.

It is in this area that Osler was truly a giant. In his work *Teacher and Student*, Osler lists four characteristics, which each student should strive for [4]. The first is the "art of detachment," or being mindful to properly balance work and play. This is not to suggest that students should not enjoy themselves. But rather that we should show self control in pursuing our delights and not allow ourselves to be overly attached to certain frivolous attractions. Osler urges that we develop a discipline of self-control so that we may live laborious days.

Second is the "Virtue of Method." Osler cites the efficiency of the successful businessman, who owes part of his success to the fact that he has developed a systematic and an orderly arrangement to his work. The best medical students and physicians I have worked with have figured this out. Some carry a notebook with them to keep track of ideas, others keep a log of outstanding tests they have ordered, but have not seen the results return yet. We healers must practice medicine under the guidelines of established system and method. This is critical to successful medical practice, but is importantly personalized by each student to their own makeup. In other words, get into the habit of doing the same thing every time, so that certain behaviors become your usual and customary practice. An example of this follows: Every time a patient tells you they have a fever, your method should be to follow this up with the question, "How high?" and if your patient reports their fever to be in the truly febrile range, e.g., over 100 degree Fahrenheit, your method should be to inquire if they have chills. And if they have chills—again—your method should dictate you to ask, "Are these shaking chills...bed rattling or teeth chattering chills?" These qualities denote rigors, a possible indicator that the patient is suffering from what may potentially be a life-threatening bacteremia. In such instances, the bacterial cell wall components are perceived as foreign by the thermoregulatory center of the brain, which responds through a cascade of signals causing the body to shake vigorously. This is an example of a good method every healer may care to follow in addressing a patient with fever. It represents a straightforward but complete process that will most efficiently lead to diagnosis and most importantly save your patient's life.

Another example of good method can be practiced every time you write a prescription. Consider lifting your head up as your pen is touching the prescription pad and ask, "Are you allergic to anything?" This simple question can quickly become extremely important if its answer is missed or overlooked. The reason being that preventable medication errors occur frequently and the last thing you (or your patient for that matter) want is the occurrence of a frightening allergic reaction on top of their current ailments. One of the greatest errors for which we are responsible for, is the inappropriate prescribing of a medication to a patient. According to the Institute of Medicine, up to 25 % of inpatients receive an incorrect medicine during their hospital stay [5]. A similar example occurs with regard to magnetic resonance imaging (MRI) scans and metal objects. It will do you well to look up each time you write an order for an MRI scan and ask your patient, "Do you have any metal inside you?" It is another simple question and often your patients will require further explanation, "Yes that includes piercings, pins, pacemakers, tattoos. . ." Unfortunately, patients have been harmed by physicians ordering an MRI without checking for metal objects. They learn this as the patient is injured during what should be a routine procedure, as the metallic particles are pulled to the surface. Sticking to this methodical series of questioning will avoid potentially uncomfortable and painful situations for those under your care.

Third is the quality of "thoroughness," knowledge of the fundamental science on which medicine is based upon. Osler instructs us to "observe, record, tabulate and communicate" and "use (our) five senses" to accomplish thoroughness. We are urged to be aware of these idealistic principles and not just attend to the minuscule details of chemistry, anatomy, and physiology. We are urged to avoid charlatanism and fraud and to study diligently the fundamentals of our discipline, so as to be truly prepared to care for our patients. A great healer, at a minimum, should be competent. With this competence must also exist the "grace of humility," the recognition that we are capable of personal error and cannot always be right; moreover, at some point we are simply going to be wrong. With every occupation come risks and consequences. If we are wrong as bakers, we may burn our rolls. But as healers, our mistakes carry a significant chance that great harm may come to our patients. An anonymous quote explains the serious truth that often "doctors bury their mistakes." Patients will die because of our mistakes, some of which may be preventable. It is our goal as healers to uphold the positive qualities explained by those before us to minimize this occurrence and to learn from any misfortune so as to prevent its reoccurrence. Osler gives advice on this as well:

> ... Errors in judgment must occur in the practice of an art which consists largely of balancing probabilities. Start, I say, with this attitude in mind, and mistakes will be acknowledged and regretted; but instead of a slow process of self-deception, with ever increasing inability to recognize truth, you will draw from your errors the very lessons which may enable you to avoid their repetition [4].

I conclude my condensed review of Osler by highlighting his success as a role model, an embodiment of the humanistic physician. Osler understood—as did all of the other physicians discussed in this book—the patient's central role in the physicians work. Osler wrote, "The good physician treats the disease; the great physician treats the patient who has the disease." This is expanded in the notion that "it is much more important to know what sort of patient has a disease than what sort of disease a patient has" [5]. Osler is often called the father of psychosomatic medicine because of his astuteness in recognizing this key concept that when it comes to helping our patients with their illnesses, one cannot separate the somatic from the psychological, the physical from the emotional, or the patient from his or her unique cultural background and life experiences. One of the more difficult challenges in medicine is care for the patient with a psychosomatic illness, especially when they possess little to no insight. Often patients and their families are in denial of or hold stigma for such illnesses, and providing your patient with proper treatment is difficult if this is the case. In situations such as this, it may be helpful to ease into education of the patient by telling them of the analogy, "The body and mind are like husband and wife, when one doesn't feel well, the other sympathizes."

Osler also urged medical students to seek a liberal education. Students of his day were urged to read for half an hour each day (in addition to their formal studies) and Osler offered the following texts as a suggested bedside library for his medical students:

Old and New Testament
Shakespeare
Montaigne
Plutarch's *Lives*
Marcus Aurelius

Epictetus
Religio Medici
Don Quixote
Emerson
Oliver Wendell Holmes – Breakfast-Table Series

Sir William Osler embodied the traits of the consummate internist, clinician, and humanistic healer. He was keenly aware of the power of observation in caring for his patients and emphasized the importance of learning from one's personal experiences. He urged the healer to develop an inner and outer calmness when approaching difficult situations and taught that by following established methods and thorough practices, we can provide the most effective care for our patients. Osler reminds us once again that patients are more than a mix of pathologic process and disease, but they are human beings who are suffering in some physical and emotional way. He advised for education of physicians in both the fields of medicine and humanities. Osler, like Hippocrates, advocated that the most successful delivery of patient care is accomplished with efforts to gain a better understanding for the *people* we strive to heal and the *artists* of medicine we wish to realize in ourselves.

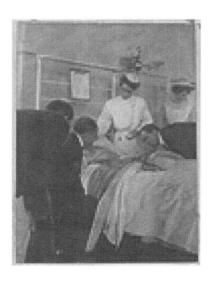

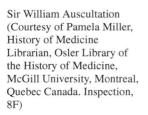

Sir William Auscultation (Courtesy of Pamela Miller, History of Medicine Librarian, Osler Library of the History of Medicine, McGill University, Montreal, Quebec Canada. Inspection, 8F)

Sir William Osler Inspection
(Courtesy of Pamela Miller,
History of Medicine
Librarian, Osler Library of
the History of Medicine,
McGill University, Montreal,
Quebec Canada.
Auscultation, 8D)

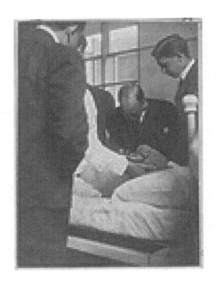

Sir William Contemplation
(Courtesy of Pamela Miller,
History of Medicine
Librarian, Osler Library of
the History of Medicine,
McGill University, Montreal,
Quebec Canada. Palpation,
8G)

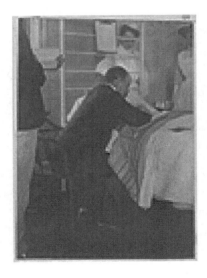

Sir William Palpation
(Courtesy of Pamela Miller,
History of Medicine
Librarian, Osler Library of
the History of Medicine,
McGill University, Montreal,
Quebec Canada.
Contemplation, 8E)

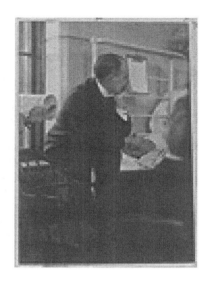

4.2 Francis Weld Peabody

"One of the essential qualities of the clinician is interest in humanity..."
–Francis Weld Peabody

Francis Weld Peabody (1881–1927) was an American medical educator. This distinguished physician was trained at Harvard and Johns Hopkins before returning to New England where he served as Professor of Medicine, Harvard Medical School; Director of the Thorndike Memorial Laboratory; and Visiting Physician and Chief of the Fourth Medical Service, Boston City Hospital. Like so many of the teachers chronicled in this text, his fame and memory—if known by those outside of academic medicine, may be best associated with a single quote—such as the one above. Peabody's adage to patient care appeared in the text *Care of the Patient*, which initially appeared in the Journal of the American Medical Association (JAMA) and later was included in a collection of Peabody's works entitled *Doctor and Patient* [6].

In *Care of the Patient*, Peabody notes that a common criticism conveyed by older practitioners is that younger graduates are overwhelmingly taught about the science of medicine, yet they lack the knowledge on how to truly *take care* of patients. The early twentieth century was a time of astounding progress and discovery in the science and technology of medicine and Peabody understood the need for teaching students of the most recent advancements. He felt that "the art of medicine and the science of medicine [were] not antagonistic but supplementary to each other," a notion that was often overpowered by the common sentiment of the time that all answers could be learned through empirical experimentation and diligent analysis. Peabody noted that part of the separation of this art from science occurs because education of early twentieth century medical students occurred solely in the hospital—a sterile, technical, dehumanizing place. This concept remains valid today. All too often hospitalized patients become identified not as who they are, but often as the disease state they represent. "That case of mitral stenosis is in the second bed on the left."

Patients are worked up scientifically, represented only by specimens and samples, histological cultures and stains; and if their extensive tests reveal an absence of physical findings or dearth of abnormal organic growth, patients may be discharged with simply, "There is nothing wrong with you." When describing inpatient medicine of his time, Peabody explained, "In hospital and in private practice... excluding cases of acute infection, approximately half of their patients complained of symptoms for which an adequate organic cause could not be discovered" [6]. However, many patients whose workups yielded negative results possessed real reasons for their sicknesses. Unfortunately for them, the most recent scientific advancements of their time produced inadequate laboratory tests by today's standards and positive results were frequently missed. Of course, those patients with functional disorders constitute a group who still require treatment. It is the medical student, Peabody notes, who is given the first opportunity to speak to the newly admitted—often lonely, frightened, stripped-naked—patient upon their admission to the hospital. The student is urged to cherish this experience and use this opportunity to form a relationship with the patient, to get to know him or her as the unique person they are.

After ruling out organic causes of ailment, we are urged to consider the prospect of functional disorder, and the best way to reveal this is by really talking to our patients. Functional disorder entails the influence of life events, emotion, mental, and psychological status of the patient and its manifestation into what seems to be physical sickness. It is recommended that the young healer make sure to investigate the life events of the patient at the time of onset of his or her symptoms. Some patients lack insight into the connection between emotional and psychological experience and the physical body. The healer may have to function as a medical detective in order to bridge the gaps to diagnosis. I once saw a recent law school graduate who complained of atypical migraine-like headaches, which appeared seemingly out of nowhere. Upon further questioning he admitted that his wife and children moved back home several states away, to give him adequate space and privacy to study for the local bar exam. Although he had agreed to this arrangement, he had not anticipated the effects it would have on his happiness and physical wellbeing. The cause of his pain was functional. The discomfort was real and its impact was profound. Peabody chooses patients with functional disorders to exemplify the profound significance of the personal relationship physicians should aim to develop with their patients, one that allows for trust between each partner and the most effective communication possible:

> The good physician knows his patients through and through, and his knowledge is bought dearly. Time, sympathy, and understanding must be lavishly dispensed, but the reward is to be found in that personal bond which forms the greatest satisfaction of the practice of medicine [5].

It is interesting to remind ourselves that earlier medical educators, such as Hippocrates, Rhazes, and Osler, also stressed the importance of functional illnesses and psychosomatic disorders and their impact on patient health. This is a common theme emphasized by many great practitioners throughout medicine. However, Francis Weld Peabody brought this idea to the forefront of medical practice during a time in which the scientific mindset dominated and technical experimentation and testing were valued perhaps more than less tangible, humanistic qualities. Peabody reminds us to be caring, thoughtful, and compassionate in dealing with our patients, to always remember that those we care for are people before they are patients. He ends his classic essay by noting something simple yet profound:

One of the essential qualities of the clinician is interest in humanity, for the secret of the care of the patient is in caring for the patient [6].

Francis Weld Peabody
(Courtesy of Boston
Medical Center)

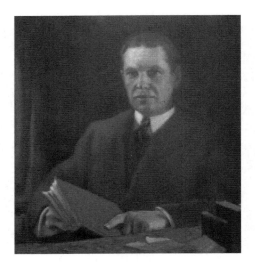

4.3 Albert Schweitzer

I do not know your destiny, but I do know one thing: the only ones among you who will be really happy are those who will have sought and found how to serve. – Albert Schweitzer

The Alsatian Lorraine theologian, physician, philosopher, and Nobel Prize winner Albert Schweitzer (1875–1965) exemplified a life committed to serving others. Like Francis Weld Peabody he was the son of a minister, born into a family that highly valued the pursuit of scholarly activities and religious study. Schweitzer received a doctorate in philosophy in 1899 and a licentiate in theology from the University of Strasbourg in 1900. By the age of 29, he was recognized as a renowned scholar in both disciplines, earning theological acclaim for his book *The Quest of the Historical Jesus*. Interestingly, Schweitzer was also an accomplished organist and earned money performing throughout Europe for much of his early life.

These funds would later be utilized to establish the jungle hospital he founded in Lambaréné, now present day Gabon. He was a musicologist as well as performer and published a biography of Johan Sebastian Bach in French in 1905, a book on organ building and playing in 1906, and rewrote the Bach book in German in 1908. Schweitzer recognized that he was born to privilege and when he was only 21 made the decision that upon turning 30 he would dedicate his life to the service of others.

Having determined to go to Africa as a medical missionary rather than as a pastor, Schweitzer began the study of medicine at the University of Strasbourg in 1905. After obtaining his MD degree in 1913, he founded the hospital that now bears his name at Lambaréné in French Equatorial Africa. In 1917 Schweitzer and his wife were sent to a French internment camp as prisoners of war. Released in 1918, Schweitzer returned to Europe and spent the next 6 years preaching in his old church, giving lectures and concerts, taking medical courses, and writing. Schweitzer published many texts including: *The Decay and Restoration of Civilization* (1923), *Christianity and the Religions of the World* (1923), *On the Edge of the Primeval Forest* (1931), and *Civilization and Ethics* (1946). Like several of the medical greats we discuss in this book, Schweitzer was an advocate for ethical behavior and service to those less fortunate. On these humanistic notions Schweitzer writes

> You ask me to give you a motto. Here it is: service. Let this word accompany you as you seek your way and your duty in the world. May it be recalled to your minds if ever you are tempted to forget it or to set it aside. Never have this word on your lips, but keep it in your hearts. And may it be a confidant that will teach you not only to do good but to do it simply and humbly. It will not always be a comfortable companion but it will always be a faithful one. And it will be able to lead you to happiness, no matter what the experiences of your lives are.

Marvin Meyer, the Director of the Albert Schweitzer Institute at Chapman University writes in his forward for *Reverence for Life: The Ethics of Albert Schweitzer for the Twenty-First Century* that Schweitzer preached how "all of us are brothers and sisters of the suffering; we all belong to each other." Schweitzer taught that we no longer belong to ourselves and that we must help those suffering, calling this the "fellowship of those who bear the mark of pain." This concept remains true today. As healthcare professionals, we are directly involved with those who suffer. We are ourselves privileged to fulfill this role, yet are also affected in some way by each healthcare interaction we experience. Every patient leaves an impression—a mark—and by taking what is important from those we provide care to, we may learn and grow as physicians. It may often seem that we belong to our patients, especially in a society in which we are sought out for specific skills, paid for service, and judged by both objective and subjective standards. However, our patients provide us service as well; the chance to learn from them, to improve our own abilities, and to provide better care in the future.

In addition to living a life of compassion and service, Schweitzer was known for his philosophy of the "Reverence for Life," which he considered to be his greatest contribution to mankind. His daughter, Rhena Schweitzer Miller is quoted as reflecting upon a conversation she had with her father one day, in which she asked him, "You have done so much for Africa. Has it given you anything in return?" He said, "Yes, nowhere else could I have found the idea of reverence for life than here" [7]. The story of how Schweitzer came upon this concept is quite interesting. In his book *Out of My Life and Thought*, Schweitzer describes how he made the conscious decision to reflect upon his personal values and understandings of the world. While taking a trip on the Ogowe River he put to words the core notions of his philosophical thought. Below is a passage that describes how he came to this revelation:

> Slowly we crept upstream, laboriously navigating – it was the dry season between the sandbanks. Lost in thought I sat on the deck of the barge, struggling to find the elementary and universal concept of the ethical that I had not discovered in any philosophy. I covered sheet after sheet with disconnected sentences merely to concentrate on the problem. Two days passed. Late on the third day, at the very moment when, at sunset, we were making our way through a herd of hippopotamuses, there flashed upon my mind, unforeseen and unsought, the phrase 'reverence for life.' The iron door had yielded. The path in the thicket had become visible. Now I had found my way to the principle in which affirmation of the world and ethics are joined together! [8]

We learn by looking at the life of Albert Schweitzer that his role as a great healer was only a part of his legendary history. He contributed as a philosopher, pastor, theologian, musician, and a prominent social activist. Schweitzer served not only people who were suffering—one patient at a time—but also mankind, as he made significant attempts to improve social health as a whole. For example, Schweitzer put forth extensive effort to immediately end atmospheric nuclear test explosions. Through careful analysis, ongoing and convincing presentation, he showed the harmful effects of radioactive fallout on humankind and the environment and he continued working to abolish the use of nuclear weapons completely. Schweitzer was given the Nobel Peace Prize in 1952, although it was withheld until Dec 10, 1953. Because of hospital duties, he was unable to come to Oslo to claim the award until 1954. His Nobel Prize speech entitled, "The Problem of Peace" [9] is considered by some to be one of the greatest speeches ever given. Part of this speech extols wealthier nations to be responsible for other nations, which were not as fortunate. "What really matters is that we should all of us realize that we are guilty of inhumanity" [7]. With the $33,000 prize money, he completed construction of the leprosarium at Lambaréné, a new facility considered so state-of-the-art that Schweitzer once said, "Now everyone is going to want to have leprosy!"

Albert Schweitzer died on Sep 4, 1965, and was buried at Lambaréné. He strongly supported the notion that one's life and practices should match their beliefs, that "a man's life should be the same as his thought." Of himself, Schweitzer confirmed, "I have made my life my argument." Perhaps the greatest lesson that healers of any age can learn from Albert Schweitzer is that we possess the potential to put our beliefs into action and that in doing so—by living in accordance with our own ideals—we may find the deepest satisfaction possible. From a practical standpoint, few, if any, of us may feel capable of leaving our current reality to travel halfway around the world and commit ourselves to our work and people in a way similar to Schweitzer. This great man found solace in commitment towards helping humankind. Although many may not fathom his decisions—i.e., practicing in a primeval forest hospital in war-torn third world countries—he teaches us that accomplishments in medicine are subjective in their affect on society and the single physician. Further, that each member of health care may find true fulfillment in their medical practice and life's work. May "everyone have his (or her) own Lambaréné."

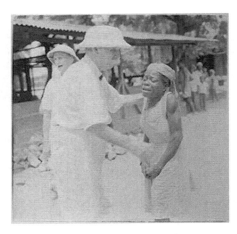

Albert Schweitzer AS-1963-343 (Schweitzer comforts a woman who was crying because others made fun of her hunched back. Courtesy of the Albert Schweitzer Fellowship Boston, Massachusetts. All photos from: The Schweitzer Album: A portrait in words and pictures by Erica Anderson, New York Harper and Row, Publishers, 1965. Reprinted with permission: Syracuse University Library, New York)

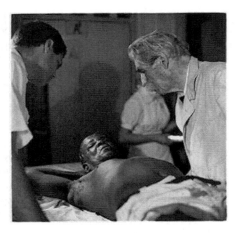

Albert Schweitzer AS-1963-526 (Schweitzer visiting a patient in the wards at his hospital. Courtesy of the Albert Schweitzer Fellowship Boston, Massachusetts. All photos from: The Schweitzer Album: A portrait in words and pictures by Erica Anderson, New York Harper and Row, Publishers, 1965. Reprinted with permission: Syracuse University Library, New York)

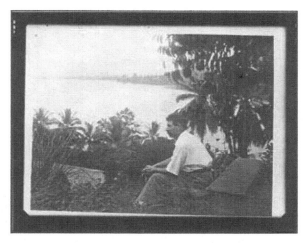

Albert Schweitzer AS-GCN-20 (Ogowe Schweitzer on the hillside near the Ogowe River at his jungle hospital during the first year. Courtesy of the Albert Schweitzer Fellowship Boston, Massachusetts. All photos from: The Schweitzer Album: A portrait in words and pictures by Erica Anderson, New York Harper and Row, Publishers, 1965. Reprinted with permission: Syracuse University Library, New York)

Albert Schweitzer by Karsh# 1 (copyright Yousuf Karsh, karsh.org)

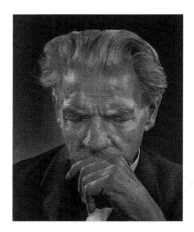

References

1. Valedictory Address to the University of Pennsylvania, 1 Mar 1989. *Aequanimatus*, 3rd Ed. New York: McGraw-Hill Inc., 1939.
2. <http://en.wikipedia.org/wiki/William_Osler>, accessed May 2009. see also: Osler Library Newsletter, no. 108, 2007 Osler Library of the History of Medicine, McGill University, Montréal (Québec) Canada http://www.mcgill.ca/files/osler-library/No1082007.pdf
3. "Preface to the Second Edition: Oxford July 1906." *Aequanimatus*, 3rd Ed. New York: McGraw-Hill, Inc., 1939.
4. "Teacher and Student." Valedictory Address to University of Minnesota, 1892. *Aequanimatus*. 3rd Ed. New York: McGraw-Hill, Inc., 1939. 23–41.
5. Institute of Medicine. Committee on Quality of Health Care in America. *To Err is Human: Building a Safer Health System*. Washington, DC: National Academy Press, 2000.
6. Peabody, F.W. *Doctor and Patient*. New York: The Macmillan Company, 1930.
7. Meyer, M.. *The Ethics of Albert Schweitzer for the Twenty-First Century: Reverence for Life*. Ed. Bergel, K.. New York: Syracuse University Press, 2002.
8. Schweitzer, A.. *Out of My Life and Thought: An Autobiography*. Trans. Antje Bultmann Lemke. New York/Baltimore: Henry Holte and Co./Johns Hopkins University Press, 1998.
9. Schweitzer, A.. "The Problem of Peace." Nobel Lecture. 4 Nov 1954.

Further Reading and Resources

Osler

The Osler History of Medicine Library at McGill University houses a tremendous number of resources, references, photos, and other links related to the works of Sir William Osler. <http://www.mcgill.ca/osler-library>

References cited by Osler History of Medicine Library include

Bliss, M. *William Osler: A Life in Medicine*. Toronto: University of Toronto Press, 1999.

Cushing, H. *The Life of Sir William Osler*. Oxford: Clarendon Press, 1925.

Osler, W. *The Quotable Osler*. Eds. Silverman, M.E. et al. Philadelphia, PA: American College of Physicians. R.R. Donnelley, 2003.

Osler, W. "Obituaries: Sir William Osler." *Br Med J* 3 Jan 1920 Vol 1.

Additional WWW sites with material by or about Sir William Osler, as suggested by The Osler Library of the History of Medicine are

Ask Osleriana—a searchable database of Osler essays

Celebrating the Contributions of William Osler, 1849–1919, an online collection of photographs, writings and letters of Sir William Osler created by the Alan Mason Chesney Medical Archives of the Johns Hopkins Medical Institution (JHMI).

Visitors to Baltimore should visit the Welch Library at JHMI and view the large painting of "The Four Greats" hanging in the second floor reading room, depicting the images of Osler, Halstead, Welch and Kelly.

Schweitzer

Schweitzer, A.. *Out of My Life and Thought: An Autobiography*. Trans. Antje Bultmann Lemke. New York/Baltimore: Henry Holte and Co./Johns Hopkins University Press, 1998.

Schweitzer, A.. *Essential Writings*. Sel. James Brazabon. New York: Maryknoll, 2005.

The Albert Schweitzer Institute

The Albert Schweitzer Institute of Chapman University is dedicated to the task of preserving, critically interpreting, and disseminating the ethical teachings of Albert Schweitzer within the context of the study of ethics and ethical values. The Institute sponsors a university course on the life and thought of Albert Schweitzer, maintains an Albert Schweitzer Exhibit on the campus of Chapman University, offers the Albert Schweitzer Award of Excellence and Schweitzer scholarships, and participates in academic programs on the legacy of Albert Schweitzer. Their website has useful and interesting information for those wanting to learn more about the life of Albert Schweitzer, and can be accessed at <www.chapman.edu/ SchweitzerInstitute>.

Another university-based website that is useful to learn more about the life of Albert Schweitzer is housed at Quinnipiac University and is accessible by visiting <www.quinnipiac.edu>.

Albert Schweitzer Nobel prize acceptance speech, "The Problem with Peace" can be read in its entirety by visiting <http://nobelprize.org/nobel_prizes/peace/laureates/1952/schweitzer-lecture.html>.

The Albert Schweitzer Fellowship sends third-year medical students to spend 3 months working as Fellows at the Albert Schweitzer Hospital in Lambaréné, Gabon, on clinical rotations. The mission of the Albert Schweitzer Fellowship is to develop "leaders in service." These are individuals who are dedicated and skilled in addressing the health needs of underserved communities and whose example influences and inspires others. More information can be obtained at <http://www.Schweitzerfellowship.org>

Schweitzer, A. *On the Edge of the Primeval Forest*. Ed. Zwischen Wasser und
    Urwald. Trans. C.T. Campion. London/New York: A. & C. Black/Holt Rine-
    hart and Winston, 1958.
My Life and Thought. Trans. C.T. Campion. London: George Allen and Unwin,
    1993; New York: Henry Holt, 1948.

Chapter 5
Modern Masters

Abstract Three physicians have been chosen from the modern era for their unique contributions to the art of medicine. Dr. Theodore Woodward, a renowned clinician-scientist, has taught the art of medicine to thousands of physicians over a career spanning decades. At the heart of his teachings has been the advice to always remember the patient in our desire to help them. Dr. Edmund Pellegrino, a bioethicist, reminds us that the physician is a moral agent who has a responsibility to be virtuous and that the good of each patient should be the goal for our actions. Dr. Paul Farmer has dedicated his life to focusing on the inequality of health care to the most vulnerable members of our society. In addition to serving the poor one patient at a time, Farmer forces us to look at the structural violence, which is disproportionately realized by the poorer and weaker members of our planet.

The lessons from these three modern masters are unified in that they call for the physician to serve our patients with humility, virtuosity, and civility. Each modern master adds to the art of medicine by way of his or her individual philosophy, his or her teachings, and as exemplified by his or her life's work.

5.1 Theodore E. Woodward

Our noble profession would be well served if the public could be made aware of its more human side.

– Theodore E. Woodward

R. Colgan, *Advice to the Young Physician*, 63
DOI 10.1007/978-1-4419-1034-9_5,
© Springer Science+Business Media, LLC 2009

Our next great teacher served at an institution very close to my heart, the University of Maryland School of Medicine. Theodore E. Woodward (1914–2005) is one of the most notable physicians to hold the position of Chairman of Medicine. Dr. Woodward received his M.D. degree from the University of Maryland School of Medicine in 1938 and became a nationally and internationally renowned authority in infectious diseases. He was instrumental in reporting the first cure for typhus and typhoid fever during World War II, which earned him a nomination for a Nobel Prize in Medicine in 1948. Dr. Woodward was acknowledged by his alma mater for undeniable dedication to teaching and commitment to patients. Over the years he received many awards, some of which include the Golden Apple Teaching Award from the University of Maryland (over a dozen times) and the Faculty Award for outstanding abilities as a teacher (over twenty times). He was a founding father of the field of infectious diseases and globally acknowledged as the premier expert on Rickettsial diseases. The details of Dr. Woodward's numerous accomplishments are not appropriate for this text, but his impact on world heath was and continues to be profound.

Aside from his great accomplishments as researcher, academician, and trailblazer in infectious disease, I have included Woodward in this book because of his contributions to the art of medicine and how he exemplified excellence by the life he chose to live. While some academic physicians climb over others to get to higher professional levels, Woodward was famous for helping others fulfill their potential. According to his longtime friend and colleague, Dr. Philip A. Mackowiak he was also generous to a fault—aiding others in their careers and research at the expense of his own accomplishments.

Dr. Mackowiak, the Chief of Medicine at the Baltimore Veterans Administration Medical Center, was himself a mentee of Dr. Woodward. Modeling his life and practice after his mentor, Mackowiak is also known by his students for his clinical astuteness, kindness, and care of the patient. Dr. Mackowiak cites a long list of physicians who were taught by Woodward and have themselves gone on to high positions of leadership. In the forward to Woodward's book *Make Room for Sentiment*, Dr. Mackowiak notes, "He will long be remembered in the minds of physicians, here and abroad, not for what he has received but for what he has contributed."

Woodward had an incredible work ethic and sense of duty to his patients. Dr. Mackowiak regularly illustrates this point to the many students rotating through the Baltimore VAMC with a story of his mentor's dedication. A prime example of this extraordinary dedication occurred one day during a Baltimore blizzard. Dr. Mackowiak recounts that as chief of medicine he felt it his duty to venture into the hospital on one particularly snowy day. He suspected that there would likely not be too much to attend to, but (just to be sure) he made his rounds as normal. This exhausting task took much longer than expected, and at the end of the day Dr. Mackowiak found himself collapsing into his chair, "head in [his] hands wondering how [he] would get home." As he looked up—much to his surprise—he saw Dr. Woodward standing in the door frame. His mentor, who was in his eighties at the time, in goulashes', a fur cap, and an old army jacket stood in front of him covered in snow and ice. It had long been known that Dr. Woodward no longer had any direct patient care responsibilities. Dr. Mackowiak wondered and inquired how it was that he arrived at the hospital? What was the purpose? Frankly, "Why are you here?" To which Dr. Woodward replied, "I hitched a ride on a snow plow." This story exemplifies the sense of duty and professionalism by which Dr. Woodward lived. This is just one example of many that illustrate this man's commitment to his profession and his patients and is one of the many reasons Dr. Woodward is regarded by Dr. Mackowiak as "my hero."

Dr. Woodward was known for his great sense of humor and his practical approach to clinical diagnosis. He would often spend over an hour with each new patient, getting to know every detail of their life story. One caution he often passed on to medical students was the warning: "Don't be a slip doctor." A "slip" is the shortened way of referring to the "lab slip," the paper form which students and house staff filled out in the pre-computer age. Dr. Woodward felt that we should sit down and talk to our patients and come to a clinical diagnosis based upon a careful analysis of the history and physical and not rely solely upon ordering laboratory tests. Perhaps Dr. Woodward's most popular proverb is the following. Recognized around the country and perhaps the world, the saying is

> If you are walking down Greene Street (the street in front of University
> Hospital in Baltimore) and you hear hoof beats behind you, don't look
> back expecting to see a zebra. Expect a horse.

In other words: common things occur commonly.

Theodore Woodward had time for anyone wanting to learn. Alas, the only personal contact I had with Dr. Woodward was when I sought his help in creating a bioterrorism presentation. I was invited by Dr. Woodward to look through his slide carousel for any slides which I might like to use for my talk. In this deck were photos he had taken during his decades of work, including documentation of those with typhus, cholera, and assorted infectious diseases. When I was invited to sit down with him, in his cluttered office down the hall from Dr. Mackowiak at the Baltimore VAMC, I truly knew that I shared company of one of the greatest physicians of our century. Dr. Woodward was careful and cautious even in his later years. True to protocol and procedure, when I offered to have all of his slides converted into digital media he turned me down saying simply, "No, it will get out of hand."

And like so many of the great teachers reviewed thus far, Woodward shares—besides of course his accomplishments as a clinician, leader, guardian of the public's health, and educator—his belief in service. In one of the many addresses he gave to the graduating students at the University of Maryland School of Medicine, Woodward made the following remarks to the class of 1983:

> Our noble profession would be well served if the public could be made
> aware of its more human side. A home visit or even a telephone call
> after a patient has been informed that he has cancer, being present dur-
> ing the time of dying or in the operating room when surgery is per-
> formed or attending a former patient's funeral serve those purposes well.
> Acceptance of these responsibilities and the discharging of them are the
> characteristics of a complete physician.

Even within a few years before his death, at the age of 91, Theodore Woodward could still be seen walking slowly down the halls of University Hospital—with his black bag in hand and a group of second-year medical students by his side.

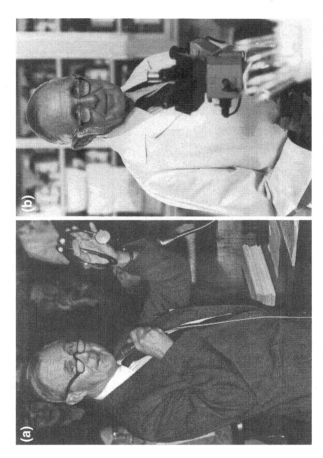

(a) Theodore Woodward (Laughing, Courtesy of Medical Alumni Association of the University of Maryland, Inc.) (b) Theodore Woodward (In front of Microscope, Courtesy of Medical Alumni Association of the University of Maryland, Inc.)

5.2 Edmund D. Pellegrino

> Do good and avoid evil is the primum principium of all ethics.
> – Edmund D. Pellegrino

One of America's greatest physician-educators in the areas of professional ethics and bioethics is Edmund D. Pellegrino. Dr. Pellegrino has been Professor Emeritus of Medicine and Medical Ethics at the Center for Clinical Bioethics at Georgetown University Medical Center since 2001. In 2004, he was named to the International Bioethics Committee of the United Nations Educational and Scientific and Cultural Organization, and in 2005 he became the chairman of the President's Council on Bioethics. Dr. Pellegrino is a prolific author and founding editor of the *Journal of Medicine and Philosophy*.

While bioethics and the philosophy of medicine may be viewed as a theoretical dilemma perhaps too overwhelming and time consuming for the busy practitioner, the Pellegrino reader comes to understand that recognition of such profound notions is as important as taking patients' vital signs. Indeed Dr. Pellegrino makes a convincing argument that the philosophy of medicine, bioethics, and the physician–patient relationship cannot be separated from one another, and in fact these exist in a very complex and entwined relationship in which each affects the other. In interviewing Dr. Pellegrino for this book, I was at first surprised when he asked *me* to define what *I* meant by the term the art of medicine, reminding me that this concept may mean different things to different people. He pointed out that the area which I seemed to be most interested in might best be described in the context of the physician–patient relationship. Dr. Pellegrino took great effort to remind me that it is this moral bond between a healer and his patient that must be cherished and safeguarded.

Many of the works of Pellegrino may prove difficult to interpret for the non-philosopher or those not fully accustomed to academic jargon. I know that I lack the educational background and knowledge base to bring the ideas of some of the great philosophers together in a manner as eloquently as he does in creating a cogent argument for his positions. Yet I immediately sat upright when I heard him speak of the "non-philosopher philosopher." I thought—that's me (and likely you). And truly this is another fantastic aspect of our vocation, the fact that we are allowed to be intimate with the human condition and invited into the lives of others. Once within this inner sanctum we are privy to things that no one else may ever know or learn. This gives every physician pause and an opportunity to speculate and admire. I believe all healers are more or less "non-philosopher philosophers," because at a minimum we *wonder*. And, according to Plato, Socrates cites in Theaetetus "all philosophy begins with wonder" [1].

It is an obvious injustice and impossibility to distill the entirety of Dr. Pellegrino's works into a few pages, and I won't. Yet if we seriously want to try to understand how to be the best healers we can, we must recognize that a significant aspect of the physician–patient relationship involves medical ethics. Dr. Pellegrino explains, "The first principle of medical ethics, the end to which it is directed, is the good of the patient." This principle can be traced back to the time of Hippocrates:

> I will follow that system or regimen which according to my ability and judgment I consider for the benefit of my patient and abstain from whatever is deleterious and mischievous [2].

In his essay *The Commodification of Medical and Health Care* [3] Dr. Pellegrino begins with a passage from *Book I of the Republic*, in which Socrates asks Thrasymachus this question:

> But tell me, your physician in the precise sense of whom you were just speaking, is he a moneymaker, an earner of fees or a healer of the sick? [4]

Dr. Pellegrino applies this notion to modern times, that today many people view our profession as having undergone a paradigm shift from a profession to a business entity. It is important to distinguish this misconception. The technician, who has learned the trade, is a member of the business community of medicine. The healer, who always keeps the patient as the center of his focus "knows the art." Physicians are often challenged to choose what is best for the patient versus what is best for the corporate bottom line. Pellegrino notes that health care cannot be a commodity, given the special nature of illness and healing [3]. We in the healing professions are afforded a special privilege by society, one that begins with the permission to learn from cadavers and extends upwards to the clinical years as we gain rudimentary skills on willing patients. Because of this special privilege, Dr. Pellegrino rightfully recognizes that we have tacitly entered into a contract with society to use the knowledge we acquire from these allowances for the benefit of those who are sick. We are urged to refrain from substituting the word "consumers" for patients or "providers" for doctors. We are urged to remain physicians and to be concerned with healing and not money-making.

There exist many instances where physicians are seduced to make more money by doing things for the patient which may be unnecessary. An example that recently came to my attention was of an ambulatory medical group that hires physicians for a base salary. The physician's income is potentially increased by incentive bonuses; which are paid out to the contractor based in part on the number of additional dollars earned through ordering in-house ancillary services and tests. This type of activity can easily be seen as encouraging, even promoting, a potential conflict of interest between what is best for the patient and what is best for the money-making physician. The physician achieves his or her bonus by ordering increased number of tests, but it is the patient who is subjected to these unnecessary tests and possibly invasive procedures. This situation just doesn't pass the sniff test: If something smells bad, perhaps it is bad.

Pellegrino feels that healers should not be gatekeepers or rationers of health care, but of course we cannot prevent this by ourselves. Society must ensure that health care does not become a commodity, and the most effective means to accomplish this is through policy, politics, and regulations. We, as physicians, possess the obligation to show them why they should put forth the effort to strive for this healthcare ideal. For society to take on this quest, we must convince our patients that we hold the faith in our profession as something sacred. If health care is "for sale" then the physician is indeed a moneymaker. Pellegrino ends his discussion on medicine as a commodity with another quote by Plato, suggesting the ethical path for all physicians, namely,

> Can we deny, then, said I, that neither does any physicians, insofar as he is a physician, seek to enjoin the advantage of the physician but that of the patient? [5]

If by reading this book your aspiration is to be best healer you can be, then as a philosopher of medicine, medical ethicist, and clinician-educator, Dr. Pellegrino will tell you that you must also recognize your role as a moral agent. On a regular basis healers must contend with certain morally questionable practices and determine how they will respond. Some specific examples include refusal to work with those who are HIV positive for fear of contagion, denying service to the poor or those with little or no insurance, cooperating with hospital authorities in discharging patients earlier than you think is reasonable, and marketing to increase the demand of dubious procedures, tests, or supplements. Pellegrino adds

> To me the most important thing in a relationship is that the heart of the relationship is a moral enterprise that occurs between not only the doctor and his patient, but the lawyer and his client, the minister and his confessor and the teacher and his student. All of these relationships have a dependent person who needs help, who goes to another person who professes to be able to help. They enter into a fiduciary relationship [6].

We are urged to be virtuous. Plato listed four cardinal virtues: fortitude, temperance, justice, and wisdom. Dr. Pellegrino, in writing of the virtues in medical practice, has extended this list to include fidelity to trust, compassion, integrity, self-effacement, and "phronesis." Phronesis is a term used by Aristotle to denote practical wisdom or the capacity for moral insight [7]. It seems reasonable that healers should strive to attain these virtues. In discussing virtue within the context of practicing medicine, Dr Pellegrino writes that virtue is aligned with excellence in living the good life:

> This excellence depends upon knowledge of good, evil, and self. It is not specialized knowledge directed to any one activity but rather to living one's whole life well. It must, like an art, be perfected through practice [8].

The virtuous physician must also be a virtuous person. This physician has character traits that define him as such and can be seen following his life according to a moral law. The virtuous physician is someone we can trust to do the right thing and to act courageously, honestly, justly, wisely, and temperately, according to Pellegrino. The virtuous physician will act well and with decent moral code even when others are not watching. While not defining the virtuous physician in specific detail, Dr. Pellegrino gives us some hints as to how he or she may be recognized. The virtuous physician is

1. A person of character—someone who can be predictably trusted to act well in most circumstances and who does not yield to the allures of power, pleasure, or self interest.
2. Someone who follows the internal morality of the (medical) profession. Profession is defined by Dr Pellegrino as "a declaration of a way of life that is specific, a way of life in which expert knowledge is used not primarily for personal gain but for the benefit of those who need that knowledge [8]."
3. Someone who practices altruistic beneficence, which implies "not only taking the interests of others into account but doing so in such fashion that our intentions and acts give some degree of preference to the intentions of others [8]."

Outwardly, the virtuous physician acting as an appropriate moral agent will exhibit behaviors characterized by fidelity to trust and promise, benevolence, effacement of self-interest, compassion and caring, intellectual honesty, justice, and prudence. Pellegrino also indicates that the virtuous physician is one who is consistent, and acts morally both at work and at home, both in professional and personal arenas, with colleagues and patients as well as family and friends. The physician's behaviors are not just seen while he or she is practicing medicine, but in all of their actions in all sections of life. Unfortunately discrepancies occur and may negatively affect one realm as expense for maintaining another. An example of such a discrepancy is the physician who is "married" to his or her work and doesn't have time for his spouse or children. A key condition of being virtuous is balancing conflicting obligations judiciously. The virtuous physician is one who acts with the "right reason," which Aristotle and Aquinas considered essential [7]. He or she realizes that they may easily be pulled in many directions by all different facets of life, but through thoughtful judgment is able to balance these opposing forces in order to achieve success in all areas. Clearly, in order to be a great healer, one must also strive to be a *virtuous* healer.

When I asked which of his many scholarly publications he considered most effective in communicating the importance of the physician–patient relationship to the young healer, who strives to be the best he or she can be with regard to the art of medicine, Dr. Pellegrino quickly cited *A Philosophical Reconstruction of Medical Morality and the Caring Ethic* [9].

In his publication, Pellegrino first describes how there exists a philosophical foundation for the obligations which bind those who profess to practice medicine, "better still, all who profess to heal [9]." He notes that today fewer physicians follow a religious foundation of ethics or remain faithful to the Hippocratic Oath. Pellegrino proposes a philosophy of the physician–patient relationship beginning with the tenet that the physician is in all aspects of life a good man or woman. Second, he explains that the nature of medicine itself is a profession—a vocation—based on healing; further, that this raises certain expectations and implies particular requirements on the part of the physician. In this essay, Pellegrino discusses Scribonius Largus, who practiced as either a physician or pharmacist—we do not know which—in the time of the Emperor Claudius. He was one of the first to refer to medicine as a vocation in the first century ACE [2]. Scribonius opined that physicians should choose to play the role required of their profession and strive to achieve the expectations implied by their position. Commiseration and humaneness are cited as unique virtues to our profession, just as truth is to a judge.

The third source of a professional basis of ethics is the physician–patient relationship itself. Throughout medical history, physicians evolved from serving as craftsman in the time of the early Greeks to being members of an elite group in society from whom patients sought care. At one point in time, physicians directed their patients like children, educated them in how to behave or care for themselves, in a true paternalistic manner. Pellegrino notes:

> Most Greek physicians in Hippocrates time were money grubbers. . .
> While at the same time there were also physicians for freemen who provided information to their patients and gave them choices. By taking the Hippocratic Oath physicians made their commitment to indicate publically that they were not among the rung of the mill practitioners. . . . This same motive was a factor in the 1847 Oath of the American Medical Association [6].

Subsequent Jewish, Christian, and Islamic religious influences, in which the self-worth of every human being is emphasized, have led to the evolution of medicine, as we know it today. Contemporary medicine is based on the development of the physician–patient relationship as a team, a partnership in which both members make decisions about the patient's individualized healthcare plan.[1] Furthermore Pellegrino argues that what the physician professes and the patient expects is a right and good healing process that is specific for each patient and their unique illnesses. Implicit in this "right and good healing process" is that the physician will be technically competent. In addition, the virtuous physician is one who insures a moral bond with their patient by providing the information necessary for the patient to make an informed decision about their care, while at the same time showing respect and consideration for the patient's wishes. If the patient cannot be his or her own advocate, then we must look to his or her surrogate (their family, guardian, or the courts) for guidance, while being as sure as possible that they do in fact have the patient's best interests at heart.

The American Medical Association (AMA) has a long history of recognizing the ethical basis of medical practice and identifies responsibility to the patient as foremost [10]. The *Principles of Medical Ethics* noted below are not laws, but standards of conduct adopted by the AMA's House of Delegates on June 17, 2001.

Principles of Medical Ethics

- A physician shall be dedicated to providing competent medical care, with compassion and respect for human dignity and rights.
- A physician shall uphold the standards of professionalism, be honest in all professional interactions, and strive to report physicians deficient in character or competence, or engaging in fraud or deception, to appropriate entities.
- A physician shall respect the law and also recognize a responsibility to seek changes in those requirements which are contrary to the best interests of the patient.

---

[1] The reader will note that many of those highlighted in this book in fact have been identified as leaders in each of their respective religious groups.

- A physician shall respect the rights of patients, colleagues, and other health professionals, and shall safeguard patient confidences and privacy within the constraints of the law.
- A physician shall continue to study, apply, and advance scientific knowledge, maintain a commitment to medical education, make relevant information available to patients, colleagues, and the public, obtain consultation, and use the talents of other health professionals when indicated.
- A physician shall, in the provision of appropriate patient care, except in emergencies, be free to choose whom to serve, with whom to associate, and the environment in which to provide medical care.
- A physician shall recognize a responsibility to participate in activities contributing to the improvement of the community and the betterment of public health.
- A physician shall, while caring for a patient, regard responsibility to the patient as paramount.
- A physician shall support access to medical care for all people.

In the *Caring Ethic*, Pellegrino further explores the evolution of the physician–patient relationship. With the introduction of scientific means of therapeutics, *curing* is indeed more prevalent; yet the *caring* aspect of health care is exceedingly neglected. The concept of care can be understood within the context of the physician–patient relationship in four ways: (1) compassion, (2) doing for others what they cannot do for themselves, (3) taking care of the medical problem, and lastly (4) "taking care" to accomplish the necessary medical protocol with conscientious attention to detail. Each physician has a moral obligation to his or her patient, and Pellegrino argues for the integration of these four elements into a unified notion of care. The following anecdote speaks to this concept.

Frank M. Calia, M.D., MACP, is Professor and Chair of the Department of Medicine, and Vice Dean for Clinical Affairs at the University Of Maryland School Of Medicine. He is a true leader in medical education, and I was fortunate to be in the audience when he spoke to an entering class of medical students on their first day of matriculation to medical school. Dr. Calia told these new medical students that in medicine there will come times when you are not sure what to do, how to proceed, or what should be done next. He then advised them to remember four simple words, "Focus on the patient." His advice reminded me of what I could imagine Hippocrates, Maimonides, Peabody, or Osler may have said as they instructed their apprentices. He further explained if you never to forget to focus on the patient, everything else will fall in proper order. This parallels Peabody's sentiment that "The secret in the care of the patient is in caring for the patient." and mirrors Pellegrino's argument for a *unified notion of care*

Pellegrino closes with a discussion defining humanistic characteristics of the medical profession. As physicians, when we are sought out to help our patients, we are professing to be competent and moreover that we will strive to use this competency to improve their total health, in all aspects of social, emotional, and physiological life. This is "a promise that we will not place our own interest first, that we will not exploit the vulnerability of those we serve, that we will honor the trust that illness forces upon those who are ill [9]." Dr. Pellegrino challenges the professed healer, the "one who declares aloud" to be mindful of and faithful to the fact that this

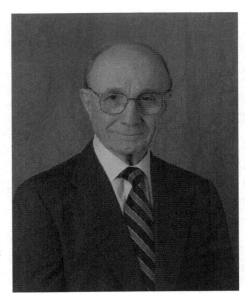

Edmund Pellegrino
(Courtesy of the American
Medical Association, as
supplied by the Presidents
Council on Bioethics)

role dictates a moral responsibility to uphold ethics in the practice of his or her art. He reminds us that the profession of medicine has its own unique philosophy which unites those who are called to this vocation and moreover that these accepted medical ethics are based upon the unique relationship between the physician and patient.

I am grateful for Dr. Pellegrino's encouragement to complete this book "Books like yours stopped thirty years ago," he told me bluntly, and this strengthened my enthusiasm as I realized he—this amazing, caring, and dedicated role model of a physician—shared my feelings for its necessity. At the end of our meeting, I was taken aback as he bid me farewell. "Be good," he whispered as we shook hands in the doorway of his office at the President's Council on Bioethics in Washington, D.C. Truly, a genuine and fitting piece of advice to come from one of the most important medical philosophers of our time.

5.3 Paul Farmer

Everyone has the right to a standard of living adequate for the health and well-being of himself and of his family, including food, clothing, housing and medical care and necessary social services, and the right to security in the event of unemployment, sickness, disability, widowhood, old age or other lack of livelihood in circumstances beyond his control.

– Universal Declaration of Human Rights, Article 25

I argue that equity is the central challenge for the future of medicine and public health.

– Paul Farmer

Paul Farmer (1959–) is a physician, medical-anthropologist, and health advocate who strongly believes the biggest challenge facing medicine in the twenty-first century is "harnessing science to help the sick and the destitute sick [11]." Farmer holds the positions of the Presley Professor of Medical Anthropology at Harvard Medical School and Chief of the Division of Social Medicine and Health Inequalities at Boston's Brigham and Women's Hospital. He is a founding director of Partners in Health, an international charity organization that provides direct healthcare services and advocates on behalf of the sick and poor. Farmer is also medical director of a charity hospital, the Clinique Bon Sauveur, in rural Haiti. His life story was superbly written and introduced to the public in *Mountains Beyond Mountains*, by Pulitzer Prize winner Tracy Kidder. Farmer is the winner of the MacArthur Foundation Genius Award and of the Margaret Mead Award for his contributions to public anthropology. He exemplifies an expert mastery of the art of medicine which is worthy of emulation. Dr. Farmer was chosen for inclusion in this book, because of the personal sacrifices he has made to serve the poor, as well as his efforts in educating others about the inequalities in housing, nutrition, and health care, which is inflicted on the destitute poor by those in power. His attention to the inequality of health care to the most vulnerable members of our society and his efforts to alleviate this disparity are nothing less than admirable.

In my mind, practicing excellence in the art of medicine by attempting to master the physician–patient relationship evokes an image of a one-to-one interaction between the healer and his or her patient. Farmer's love and concern for his individual patients is detailed beautifully in Kidder's book, including the care he has provided not only to the poor in Haiti over the past twenty years but also to those in Peru, the Soviet Union, South America, and elsewhere. It may seem unusual to include Paul Farmer in a book with purpose to educate young physicians on how to transition from technician to healer based on his fame, but it is the precise manner in which he did so that makes him even more noteworthy. This mentor gained his fame not by seeking it, but by purely promoting a better way of providing health to an underserved subsection of society— those who are without the basic necessities which are assumed, even expected, to be available in many parts of the world. Farmer argues that "Anyone who wishes to be considered humane has ample cause to consider what it means to be sick and poor in the era of globalization and scientific advancement [11]." This is in stark contrast to those who must suffer through illness in areas of the world without access to appropriate care or those willing to help. We are given many examples to consider in any one of his several of books (see additional reading below).

Farmer's *Pathologies of Power: Health, Human Rights, and the New War on the Poor* won the 2006 J.I. Staley Prize for outstanding work in anthropology. In his text, the physician–anthropologist reveals that the most basic of human rights—the right to survive— is being denied to the most vulnerable of our world's population. Freedom from want is the human right most applicable, and unfortunately most denied, to many of his patients. Physicians of course need access to medicines and supplies to physically practice medicine, yet he challenges us to be more active in social and economic rights as a logical extension in care of the patient. The fact that this rhetoric comes from someone who has witnessed this inequality first-hand makes his story all the more compelling. Farmer's life story, like so many of those described in this book, is what provides the human experience and foundation for his argument. He has travelled to the poorest communities on the planet and lived side by side with those he serves. Whereas humanism advocates for focusing on the individual, Farmer might argue that you must not forsake the public health of a community for the individual patient. As physicians, we are responsible to both the individual and society, and although this relationship sometimes manifests in dilemma it should never be far from the physician's mind. He would certainly proclaim that the rich and powerful—or perhaps the physician who exists in a relatively powerful role in relation to the relatively vulnerable patient—must not forsake the poor and weak. His call for involvement in the bigger, global manner of advocating for equitable health care for those who cannot effectively speak for themselves cannot be rebutted by a true healer. In fact, it must be a principle by which the true healer lives his or her life.

In *Pathologies of Power*, Farmer describes in detail the many ways that the powerful take advantage of the poor. Examples of such abuses include "the cruel and unusual punishment" which is inflicted upon prisoners who suffer from tuberculosis in many parts of the world. The cruelty manifests as inmates are denied proper medical care, which leads to an unavoidably increased morbidity and mortality that these people experience. The high rate of this occurrence is alarming. We learn that TB transpires in prisons at rates 5 to 10 times the national average. And with increasing rates of TB evolves the extremely treatment-resistant strains. Drug-resistant tuberculosis is viewed therefore as a special form of punishment for these inmates, as they must suffer through progression of a more intense and life-threatening illness than a person given proper care. Farmer and his colleagues were invited to the Soviet Union as TB specialists in an effort to help curb this disease, which at the time was the number one cause of death in Soviet prisons. The group worked to not only improve the health for the individual patients but also improve the prisons and society as a whole. Overcrowding, poor ventilation, a lack of financial resource allocation to treat multi-drug-resistant strains are but a few of the reasons for this epidemic. Farmer calls for protective public policies to help those who are victimized by this inhumane treatment. Furthermore he warns, "Transnational TB epidemics will at least remind the affluent few that as long as those epidemics remain out of control, no one is really safe [12]."

Like Edmund Pellegrino, Paul Farmer conveys how "the commodification of medical care is one of the biggest human rights issues facing the 'modern' world today [13]." When the term "patient" is substituted by "clients" we see the commercialization of health care and the shift of the physician from healer to service-provider. Farmer notes that clients (not patients) indeed are customers, someone who pays for their services. When they are viewed as such the service in question is being defined as a commodity and not a right. Farmer is obviously repulsed by such a notion and provides many specific examples as to how this occurs, such as the fact that cancer care is almost unknown among the world's bottom billion. Farmer tells the story of one woman who was rescued from breast cancer by his organization, Partners in Health, as society turned its shoulder and otherwise left her to die from her disease. He details the story of an impoverished Haitian woman who was fortunate to undergo a mastectomy by a volunteering Cuban surgeon. Bridging resources across the globe, she was able to subsequently have her cancerous growth analyzed by pathologists at Brigham Women's Hospital and received chemotherapy donated by benefactors. This woman survived because of the efforts of Farmer and his colleagues as they reached above and beyond to bring her in contact with the necessary care.

To highlight the exceptional care provided by Partners in Health in Haiti, a photographic exhibit called "Structural Violence: A View From Below" was shown in Boston a few years back. One of the exhibit's guests expressed her displeasure with a photo taken by Dr. David Walton of this same poor woman, who was shown bare-chested to reveal an extensive left mastectomy scar. The entry in the guest book read, "Not appropriate at all." Farmer tells of the strife that many impoverished people undergo in the struggle to access needed health care, which is often only overcome by those with financial resources. He notes that the comment in the guest book speaks to an instinct that many in our society possess, which is to avert our gaze from things that make us uncomfortable. The guest's comment conveys an honest but unfortunate misunderstanding of intention and focuses on a superficial display of "inappropriateness" rather than seeing the beauty in this woman's survival—the fact that so many resources came together through the work of these physicians and overcame societal shortcomings to save her and others like her. Farmer concludes:

> Those who must face structural violence every day encounter precious little in the way of support for the right to food, water, housing or medical care. . .. We need to rehabilitate a series of sentiments long out of fashion in academic circles: compassion; indignation on behalf not of oneself but of the less fortunate; empathy; and even pity [14].

I initially hesitated in extending beyond discussions of the traditional physician–patient relationship to recognize a respected belief of the physician's duty to society; however, I feel it is extremely important to acknowledge Farmer's call for the promotion of public health improvement. Further, it is clear that great physicians through the ages are of the same opinion. We cannot relegate our duty to our patients at large. Particularly in this age of globalization, we are more easily connected to those who are in need of health care throughout the world, and thus our ideal goals of improving social and global health are indeed reachable in a way that they were not for many centuries. I pursue a call for greater advocacy for those who are victims of inequality of health care—but do not feel intimidated reader. I do not think that anyone of us should feel guilty for practicing "conventional medicine" and serving our patients faithfully in areas where access to health care is better than other parts of the country or world. I do, however, think we are challenged to face the harsh reality that there are many others who are not getting the care they deserve and that perhaps we can do more to alleviate this disparity. Despite many advancements in medical and communication technology, this is still no easy task. I do not suggest that in order to be a consummate healer you should be willing to relocate to another country, as Schweitzer and Farmer have done. I am encouraged with the wisdom of Schweitzer who as noted previously

Dr. Paul Farmer
(Courtesy of Gilles
Peress, as supplied by
Partners in Health
/Harvard Medical School,
Boston, MA)

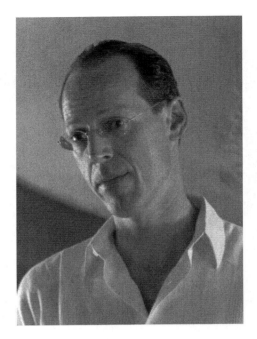

cited that anyone can "have a Lambaréné." The truth is, you are
needed right where you are called to be.

References

1. Plato: Theaetetus (Focus Philosophical Library), Joe Sachs, R Pullins Co.
   Mar 2004.
2. "The Oath." *The Genuine Works of Hippocrates*, Trans. Francis Adams.
   Baltimore, MD: Williams and Wilkins, 1939.
3. Pellegrino, E.D. The Commodification of Medical and Health Care: The
   Moral Consequences of a Paradigm Shift from a Professional to a Market Shift. *The Philosophy of Medicine Reborn A Pellegrino Reader*. Eds.
   Engelhardt, H. Jr. et al., Notre Dame, IN: University of Notre Dame Press,
   2008. 101.
4. Plato. *Republic*. 341c.
5. Plato. *Republic*. 342c.
6. Personal communications with Dr. Edmund Pellegrino, Jul 2008.
7. Pellegrino, E.D. *The Virtues in Medical Practice*. Oxford: Oxford University Press, 1983.

8. Pellegrino, E.D. "Character, Virtue and Self Interest in the Ethics of the Profession." *The Philosophy of Medicine Reborn A Pellegrino Reader*. Eds. Engelhardt, H. Jr. et al., Indiana: University of Notre Dame Press, 2008. 135.

9. Pellegrino, E.D. and Thomasma, D.C. . *A Philosophical Basis of Medical Practice, A Philosophical Reconstruction of Medical Morality*. Oxford: Oxford University Press, 1981.

10. "Principles of Medical Ethics." American Medical Association. Jun 2001. 10 Apr 2009. <http://www.ama-assn.org/ama/pub/physician-resources/medical-ethics/ama-code-medical-ethics/principles-medical-ethics.shtml>.

11. "Review of Lecture by Dr. Paul Farmer." Harvard Public Health Now. 17 Sep 2004. 29 Mar 2009. http://www.hsph.harvard.edu/now/sep17/program.html>.

12. Farmer, P.. *Pathologies of Power: Health Human Rights, and The New War On The Poor*. Berkeley, CA: University of California Press, 2005. 195.

13. Lipsiae. *Remedies*. Eds. S. Largus et al., 1887.

14. Farmer, P.. "Suffering That is 'Not Appropriate at All,'" *Revista,* 2003, 3: 42–47.

Further Reading and Resources

Pellegrino, E.D. and Thomasma, D.C. , *A Philosophical Basis of Medical Practice*. Oxford: Oxford University Press, 1981.

Pellegrino, E.D. *Humanism and the Physician*. Knoxville, TN: The University of Tennessee Press, 1979.

Pellegrino, E.D. *The Virtues in Medical Practice*. Oxford: Oxford University Press, 1983.

Kidder, T.. *Mountains Beyond Mountains: The Quest of Dr. Paul Farmer, A Man Who Would Cure The World*. New York: Random House Trade Publications, 2004.

Farmer, P. *Pathologies of Power: Health Human Rights, and the New War On The Poor*. Berkeley, CA: University of California Press, 2005.

Farmer, P. *Infections and Inequalities: The Modern Plagues*. Berkeley, CA: The University of California Press, 1999.

Farmer, P. *The Uses of Haiti*. Common Courage Press, 1994.

Farmer, P. *AIDS and Accusation: Haiti and the Geography of Blame*. California Series in Public Anthropology. Berkeley, CA: The University of California Press, 1992.

Resources

Information on Partners in Health, Boston, MA, can be found at www.pih.org.

Chapter 6
Survival Tips for the Young Physician

Abstract Practical advice for the young physician is offered in this chapter. How to effectively present a patient is a critical talent, which all artists of medicine should have. Succinct directives are given on how to convey medical information with clear examples so that the reader may easily understand what is expected of them. The young physician is taught that the best way to get better at the practice of medicine is to see more patients, while learning from each one. You will be let in on a truism in medicine that is rarely discussed: all great clinicians started out in their careers just as you are doing—young, green, and inexperienced. Good communication techniques are highlighted. A simple mnemonic is reviewed which will help every reader focus on how to best show that the care of the patient intended is communicated effectively.

6.1 The Art of Presentation

The skill of presentation is fundamental to practicing the art of medicine. It is important to effectively convey the logic behind your actions, whether in writing or oral presentation. I repeatedly see students, residents, and even physicians present in a haphazard way. These people often have intelligent contributions to make to discussion, but often their message is lost in confusion and disarray of ideas. In this section, I aim to underscore some of the crucial

R. Colgan, *Advice to the Young Physician*,
DOI 10.1007/978-1-4419-1034-9_6,
© Springer Science+Business Media, LLC 2009

elements of a good presentation, so that others will appreciate how truly gifted you are.

You should begin by understanding what is expected of you, to know the basics about what factual information must be conveyed in this exchange. It is equally as important to know who will be the recipient of your message, as well as what specific format they prefer. A presentation to a cardiologist will not be the same as a presentation to an obstetrician by nature of their professional differences. Be sure you know the parlance of each specialty and what is typically looked for by different specialists. For instance, when presenting patient information to a cardiologist, you must be sure to know all the coronary artery disease (CAD) risk factors of your patient, as well as previous cardiac catheterization details. If your patient has chest pain, be sure to include the descriptors of angina too. An obstetrician is going to want to know your patient's last menstrual period, menstrual cycle characteristics, and gestational history. Regardless of the specialty, there are some critical facts that must always be accounted for and reported. Look to understand upfront if you are being asked to give a full comprehensive presentation, e.g., a formal morning report or if a one-minute, "tell me who you admitted last night" description is expected.

Young healers typically get a brief rundown on how to properly present a patient and are encouraged to describe this information in a certain order. Often this education is inadequate, and they learn shortly after how they screwed something up—how they should have put this in the history of present illness (HPI) or left something else out of the analysis, etc. It is important to learn how to present a patient efficiently and thoroughly for three reasons. First, if you follow Osler's admonition of developing a particular method, you will consciously do things the same way each time and are less likely to forget something of significance. If you always order your presentation as chief complaint, history of present illness, past medical history, current medications then allergies, you are less likely to ever forget to ask your patient if they are allergic to something and even less likely to prescribe a medicine that may result in a fatal allergic reaction. Implicit for a good presentation is that you have performed your evaluation in a thorough manner and that you have followed a proper method. For example, present the history with proper method by recounting the patient's story in a chronological and descriptive manner. Present the physical exam with proper method by logically displaying information from head to toe.

Second, it is important to present effectively so that your listener, typically a fellow clinician, can clearly understand what you did or plan to do. A good presentation will enable a subsequent care provider to easily pick up where you left off and provide a smooth transition to enable the best possible patient care. A good presentation is not a comprehensive data dump, where you look to impress the listener with the fact that you asked everything. A good presentation is giving the listener the significant information they need to know so as to be able to understand what you learned, have input into the case, and perhaps eventually take over that person's care. An example of an improper patient presentation is calling your attending at two in the morning to give an overly thorough description of your stable patient's entire health history including his banana allergy. (This actually happened to me!) You should succinctly give your listener the information they need to make their own independent assessment as to what is going on with the patient. This part is slightly tricky, because it implies that you know all of the pertinent positive and negative questions and answers to include in your presentation—which as a young healer you may not. You are learning these as you pursue your training and will continue to learn more and more each day of your career. Like any other skill, the discovery and recognition of significant information comes with practice.

Third, you should strive to learn how to present well, because it is the language of medicine. The listener is often going to evaluate and assume your competence based in part on how well you use the language of medicine—in short, how well you presented. To be blunt, you can be brilliant, yet present badly, and your mentor will think you to be disorganized or incompetent. The sooner you master the skill of presentation, the sooner you will impress all of those who listen to you and earn recognition as someone who is organized and coherent. You will more likely be viewed as competent. Let me go over a few rules:

In giving a presentation you simply start at the beginning, which is always the chief complaint. This is best given in the patient's own words and not your assessment of what they meant. In other words, say that the patient stated, "I couldn't breathe" rather than, "The patient presented with shortness of breath or dyspnea." The chief complaint is always followed by the history of present illness

(HPI). This is the most important part of the entire history, so you want to be very careful that you attend to it well. Begin by describing the patient, e.g., "This is the first university hospital admission for this 24 year old African American female who was last well until the evening prior to admission when she noted she couldn't breathe." The HPI should read like a newspaper article, wherein the most important sentence—or the lead—is first and then subsequently followed then by more detailed information of lesser importance. Like a good journalist, do not bury your lead! Do not hide a critical piece of historical information further down in the body of the report, when in fact it is crucial to understanding the patient's illness. For instance, if your patient was also suffering from an underlying malignancy, was on oral contraceptive therapy, and her shortness of breath occurred simultaneously with the abrupt onset of a dry cough, on the day after her long airplane flight, which was one week after she had her left leg placed in a cast for a chip fracture of the ankle that occurred while skiing, say so. She may have a pulmonary emboli, and as you present your patient in a logical and prioritized fashion, you will help your colleague better understand how you achieved that conclusion. Although each piece of information could theoretically be categorized under many different parts of the patient's history, they are details that are extremely important in deciphering the case. It is up to you to recognize them as such and give them to your listener as coherently and concisely as possible.

In your HPI present your data methodically, chronologically, in a continuum from when the patient felt well, to the present sick condition. Follow your HPI with past medical history, medications, and allergies. For example, "The patient is allergic to codeine and suffered anaphylactic shock when she took it in the past." Even if a nurse or medical assistant has filled this information in for you, you should personally ask each patient about medications and allergies. Do this every time you see a patient, for the rest of your life. To not do so is bad practice, and mistakes made by missing this opportunity to collect and/or confirm valuable patient information can harm your patient and your career. We will talk about choosing good practice later on. This is a good template for the most essential components of the subjective portion of your presentation. Remember to collect as much information as possible. If asked, you should be prepared to provide supplemental facts from the family history, social history, and review of systems, while realizing that pertinent information should already have been mentioned in the HPI.

The objective exam should always begin with your patient's general appearance followed by his or her vital signs. The general appearance should be such that you could easily pick the patient from a crowd of people or a waiting room. Remember that the vital signs are ... vital. In fact they are arguably, along with the general appearance, the most important signs under the objective portion of your presentation. Yet these two descriptors are often given little to no mention. You can be brief in saying that your patient "looks to be in no acute distress and is with stable vital signs," just be sure to include some recognition of this valuable information. Also, as with the history of present illness, make sure to mention significant vital signs when they apply directly. If our theoretical patient was suffering from a pulmonary emboli, we would want to specifically mention her respiratory rate and if she appeared to be in any respiratory distress. Almost every patient you care for in the clinical practice of medicine, certainly in primary care medicine, should have his or her heart and lungs auscultated. Granted, there may be some particular exceptions to this rule; but most physicians should listen to their patient's heart and lungs at each visit. This is not necessarily for the purpose of discovering some pathology—not to search for a mid systolic click or pick up subtle bronchophony—but so you may lay your hands on the patient. Every great healer knows the value of (appropriately) touching your patient. You should go out of your way to practice a "laying on of the hands." It is part of a therapeutic, professional intimacy between physician and patient, a conveyance of compassion for the person you are providing care. It is a sign, at a minimum, of *kindness*. Lastly, be sure to comment on "the other" or anything else in the physical exam that may be noteworthy. In our patient above, you may also comment that you do or do not hear a fixed splitting of the second heart sound as might be heard in massive pulmonary emboli.

After your objective exam comes the hardest part for the young healer: the assessment and plan. It is the most challenging, for the less clinical training you have experienced the less ability you possess to develop a broad differential diagnosis. The assessment should not be a repetition of your history and physical. It should be your synthesis of a working diagnosis, even if you do not know what is going on. Continuing our example: If you are not sure what is causing your patient's shortness of breath, you should list what you know as fact: "Problem number one is dyspnea, etiology unclear. Problem number two is recent left leg fracture. Problem number three is previous codeine anaphylaxis, and problem number four is health maintenance—it is noted that it has been several years since her last pap smear." Call your patient's problem what you understand it to be at the time. Other examples might be "chest pain, etiology unclear" or "vesicular unilateral T5 dermatomal eruption, etiology unclear." By stating your working diagnosis, you know where you are and are given a lead as to how to proceed. Also, it communicates to your listener that the gears are turning, and you are thinking along a logical train of thought, even if you have not yet arrived at the answer.

Lastly is your plan. This plan should be congruent with your assessment. If you have mentioned three active problems in your assessment, you should have three active plan items. The plan also includes patient education goals, prescription of medications, and diagnostics including any additional studies you would like to order. In addition, every time you see a patient it is wise to include in your plan what they can do to help themselves, as well as when they should contact you again and return for care. Some variations to this apply. If you are seeing a patient for an acute or sick visit, there should be some mention of health maintenance under his or her assessment or plan. This is your opportunity to inquire if they are up to date on their age-appropriate health screening, e.g., an annual well-woman exam. If not, part of your plan should be a recommendation that your patient also consider making an appointment for whatever health screening exams they require. In continuing with the example of our clinical case of a young woman with shortness of breath, our plan might have the following components: "(1) Explained to patient my concern for a life threatening pulmonary emboli; she agrees to emergency department transfer by ambulance for consideration of imaging studies to rule out pulmonary emboli; (2) Continued non weight bearing and use of crutches in light of her recent leg fracture; (3) Avoid codeine given allergy to same; consider non steroidal anti-inflammatory for pain relief; and (4) Patient urged to make a follow up visit, at a later

date for a well woman exam." One of my partners in private practice taught me that in his residency they encouraged physicians to
include under plan, in addition to what was discussed above, any recommendations about diet, exercise, and stress. Hippocrates would
be proud.

Common mistakes occur as presentations become disorganized
and messy. Your presentation should start with the subjective
("S" What did your patient say?) followed by the objective ("O"
What did you observe, auscultate, palpate, percuss... find?), followed by your assessment ("A" What do you think is going on?)
and finally your plan ("P" What are you going to do?) A common
mistake that all new clinicians make is going from topic to topic, or
from "S" to "P" to "A" to "O" to "S" to "O" to "S" again, back to
"P" followed by ... etc. My advice to you is: to tell them the S, the
pertinent "S" and nothing but the "S." Then pause. Indent your presentation so the listener knows you are now leaving "the land of S,"
for the "land of O." When you get to "O," always begin with general
appearance, followed by those most vital signs. When young healers get to the assessment they often want to repeat the "S" and "O"
again. You must fight hard not to do this and continue on to "A" and
"P" by lying out the patient's problems and attempted solutions. My
advice to the young healer is to practice your presentation skills as
often as you can and be thankful when a senior clinician "pokes you
in the ribs" and tells you to do it differently. You must always strive
to be the best communicator of medicine possible. In the end, the
patient will be better served and you will be a better physician.

6.2 Practice Makes for Better Practice

A common lament of the younger physician is the misunderstanding that you have to know it all. Even the best-seasoned
clinicians start out young, green, naïve, with little clinical experience. When I chose to go into private practice, I specifically
sought out a group of several doctors older than myself thinking that I would be able to learn from them. I was not disap-
pointed. But even then I did not know how much I didn't know.
I was surprised when the venerable and wise senior physician
of our group told me shortly after my arrival, "Don't worry in

about 10 years you'll get in your groove." I was astounded to think that it would take 10 years. But he was right, i.e., the longer you practice medicine, the better you get at it. Another academic physician who had been practicing for 25 years told me of being urged by his wife to give up obstetrics. When asked why he decided to stay in the field he reasoned, "I am just getting good at it."

The young healer must understand that you are not required to know it all, during your studies, upon graduation from medical school, or even through residency. But once you are practicing on your own, you are responsible for knowing what you know and being humble enough to acknowledge what you do not know in order to practice the standard of care. One of the best skills to develop as a young healer is the capacity to say, "I don't know." After which of course must follow the conscious reflection of evaluating the situation and deciding how next to proceed. This may seem difficult on the surface, but really simplifies to the question of whether or not the given situation, in the clinical area you are unfamiliar with, is or is not an emergency? If you come upon a victim of a motor vehicle accident on the side of the road and blood is shooting from his carotid artery: apply compression. This is an emergency! If it is an emergency— or the patient's airway, breathing, or circulation is compromised— call for immediate help. Short of situations as dire as this, most everything else is either urgent or elective. Urgent matters can be clarified by talking with a colleague, picking up the phone, referring to a textbook, or looking something up on the internet. An urgent clinical issue implies that if you do not attend to the matter promptly harm may be done to the patient. In the earlier clinical case scenario, the young female patient who presented to the ski patrol with a painful swollen ankle (and not yet with chest pain or shortness of breath) could be categorized as someone in need of urgent care. She should have her ankle problem addressed promptly. As opposed to urgent problems, elective problems can generally wait a while to be attended to. Elective clinical problems are those in which you are unsure of how to next proceed, and these can typically wait until you obtain the information you need to make an appropriate decision. A decision to start a cholesterol-lowering agent in a patient for whom you are unclear as to the proper application of the latest recommendations for drug interactions can wait until you have the chance to check the literature.

In researching for this book I spoke to many physicians and contacted colleagues who I personally hold in high esteem to gain their insights on the art of medicine. I asked them who they considered exemplary figures throughout medical history, those who practiced the art of medicine in a manner to which we all should aspire to. Many shook their heads and let their voices trail off after naming only one or two figures. But when I asked how it was they learned the art of medicine, most replied that the greatest lessons came from working alongside a revered mentor. Although lessons on the art of medicine as taught by "ordinary healers" is not the theme of this book, the truth is that all of us look to role models for the types of behavior we want to emulate. This modeling of good practices is one of the most important ways we learn the art of medicine. We practice it and inspire those around us to do the same. "The Practice of Medicine is an art based on a science," Osler tells us. It entails skills and crafts that we learn from seeing others do it. "See one, do one, teach one" is an adage that most interns have heard. This applies not only to procedure—directing how to put in an intravenous line or drain an abscess—but also to many of the softer, subtler ways that physicians practice their craft, their *art*.

When I was a third-year resident I remember doing a rotation with Dr. J Roy Guyther in Mechanicsville, Maryland. Dr. Guyther is one of Maryland's giants in family medicine, who helped develop the specialty from the horse and buggy general practitioner to the current residency-trained family physician. I did not expect to learn so much about evidence-based medicine and the art of its practice from my grey-haired mentor, and I am fortunate to have shared many experiences with him. I recall one memorable moment in particular: I was watching Dr. Guyther help an elderly woman on a particularly busy afternoon. She arrived with a litany of complaints, all of which he addressed, and this caused him to be even further behind then he already was. Thinking the extended visit was finally over, he walked toward the door. The patient said, "Dr. Guyther, there is. . . one more thing." "What is that," he replied, to which she answered "I'd like to talk to you about my constipation." I never expected what happened next. Dr. Guyther returned to his seat and over the next several minutes he actually took the time to listen to her concerns, ask more details and help her with her problem. These "oh by the way" questions, also known as the "hand on the door knob" concerns, occur quite often and can be a significant source of stress for the physician as they are interpreted as an inconvenience or obligation. Often, if physicians do not take the time to address these concerns, the patient interaction is rushed and incomplete. But in this situation, Dr. Guyther modeled for me, considerate patient care, and this has been just as significant in my medical education as those who have shown me the proper procedure to obtain an arterial blood gas. Although the time for this assistance was not in his schedule, Dr. Guyther made the time because the patient needed him. He selflessly attended to his patient and provided her with exceptional care.

These instances of phenomenal patient care can be as simple as the one above or may be life-altering. Dr. Edward Kowalewski, one of the founding fathers of the American Academy of Family Physicians and the first Chair of the Department of Family and Community Medicine at the University of Maryland, proved that taking the necessary time to provide thorough and expert care can truly change the patient's life. A patient once sought Dr. Kowalewskis' help in an office visit, during which he disclosed that he had just killed another man. As the story goes, Dr. Kowalewski installed a switch that could be activated from his exam room desk, which turned on a "do not disturb" red light outside the room. Ninety minutes after having indicated that he did not want to be interrupted during this patient visit, the two men emerged from the consultation and walked to the police station, where the patient turned himself into authorities. Observing "ordinary" healers doing extraordinary things for their patients is how many seasoned clinicians describe their experience of learning the essentials of the physician–patient relationship. We learn to be better healers not only through diligent study and committed practice but by seeking out mentors and striving to model exceptional behaviors. I hope that the value of this book is evident as it recognizes some of these behaviors and examples set by many who are no longer here to teach us. Their lessons have withstood the test of time and should not be forgotten.

6.3   Good Communication

Communication is an essential skill required for any person with ambitions to become a great healer. One of the leading reasons why patients complain about their doctors is a lack of explanation and poor communication [1]. Poor communication between the physician and patient has been shown to be a factor in malpractice litigation [2]. So while hopefully we can agree that good communication is necessary and valuable, this begs the question: How can we learn how to better communicate with our patients? We all think we know good communication when we hear it, but how do you practice it?

In May 1999, 21 leaders and representatives from major medical education and professional organizations attended an invitational conference in Kalamazoo, Michigan, with the goal of delineating a coherent set of essential elements in physician–patient communication [3]. The participants wanted to devise a short list of elements to characterize effective communication, provide tangible examples of skill competencies that would be useful to medical educators at all levels and be both evidence-based and amenable to assessment and evaluation. The end product of the Bayer-Fetzer Conference on Patient–Physician Communication in Medical Education is summarized below.

The Kalamazoo Consensus Statement

Essential Elements of Communication in Medical Encounters

1. *Build a relationship*: Develop a patient-centered or relationship-centered approach to care. Strive to build a partnership with your patient, while realizing that the patients ideas and values maybe different than your own.
2. *Open the discussion*: Hear what the patient has to say in his or her own words, attempting to understand what they may be worried about, while making a connection with your patient.
3. *Gather information*: Use open-ended and closed-ended questions to better understand what is going on; trying to clarify what you

need to know and summarizing what you think you understand, while actively listening to the patient using non-verbal and verbal techniques.

4. *Understand the patient's perspective*: Try to understand your patient's background better, e.g., family, cultural, socioeconomic, and spiritual, inquiring as to his or her beliefs and concerns and what they hope to achieve from his or her visit with you.

5. *Share information*: Be sure that you are communicating with your patient in a manner that they can easily understand, e.g., avoiding medical terminology that may be misunderstood and being mindful of his or her educational background. Afterwards the committee advises checking back with your patient to see if they understood what you were trying to convey and if they had any additional questions.

6. *Reach agreement*: Develop a consensus between you and your patient as to how you will both proceed, while enlisting resources and supports that may help you both.

7. *Provide closure*: And lastly determine if your patient has any additional concerns, summarizing what you understand to be your conjoint plan and discussing when you should meet again.

Gregory Makoul, Ph.D., Chief Academic Officer and Senior Vice President for Innovation and Quality Integration at St. Francis Hospital in Hartford, Connecticut, provided leadership in writing the Kalamazoo statement and has also offered another article containing a mnemonic that some may find helpful in remembering some of the above techniques [4]. The SEGUE framework for teaching and assessing communication skills stands for: *S*et the stage, *E*licit information, *G*ive information, *U*nderstand the patient's perspective, and *E*nd the encounter.

Good communication and clinical judgment are critical talents for the aspiring healer to achieve. You may have a brilliant intellect, effectively practice evidence-based medicine, and show great consideration for your patient. But if you cannot clearly and efficiently convey your clinical impression to a colleague or your patient you will be undervalued and the physician–patient relationship will not nearly be as rich or satisfactory. Presenting a patient properly, effectively communicating with your patient, and maintaining sound clinical judgment are talents which we are not born with, but must learn and develop over time. If you feel like you are not where you want to be in this regard, that is a good sign. It means you recognize that you can do better—and you will. Throughout your transition from technician to healer, keep in mind that every mentor you have ever looked up to, every person you view as being exemplary in the practice of medicine began his or her clinical career as a young physician just like you.

References

1. Vincent, C., et al. "Why Do People Sue Doctors?" *Lancet* 1994, 25 Jun, 343:1609–1613.
2. Beckman, H., Markakis, K., Suchman, A.L. , Frankel, R. . "The Doctor-Patient Relationship and Malpractice: Lessons from Plaintiff Depositions." *Arch Intern Med* 2000, 154: 1365–1370.
3. Participants in the Bayer-Fetzer Conference on Physician-Patient Communication in Medical Education. "Essential Elements of Communication in Medical Encounters: The Kalamazoo Consensus Statement." *Acad Med* 2001, 76(4): 390–393.
4. Makoul, G. "The SEGUE Framework for Teaching and Assessing Communication Skills." *Patient Educ Couns* 2001, 45(1): 23–24.

Further Reading and Resources

How To Present

A guide to improving presentation of oral cases can be found at the site below:

<http://depts.washington.edu/medclerkhj/student/presentation.html>

In addition, Loyola University provides an instructional video about "Oral Presentation on Rounds," accessible below:

<www.medicalvideos.us/play.php?vid=740>

Practice Makes for Better Practice

Selzer, R. *Letters to a Young Doctor*. Boston, MA: Mariner Books, 1996.
Groopman, J. *How Doctors Think*. Boston, MA: Mariner Books, 2008.

Chapter 7
Civility

Abstract Patients want their doctors to be polite and civil as well as competent. Tips on how to practice etiquette-based medicine, as advanced by Dr. Michael Kahn, are presented. Expanding on this concept is a look at the 25 rules of civil conduct authored by Dr. P.M. Forni. Specific examples of how these rules of conduct may be incorporated into our clinical practice are discussed.

A healer must uphold a professional, considerate, and kind manner during all interactions with his or her patients. This notion applies from the time of introduction and initial exam, through follow-up consults, visits with family members, and any other patient encounter. Hippocrates explains how a physician should compose himself or herself from the very moment they meet the patient. In *Decorum*, we are taught upon entering a patient's room to "bear in mind [our] manner of sitting, reserve, arrangement of dress, decisive utterance, brevity of speech, composure, bedside manners, (and) care [1]." Dr. Michael W. Kahn, a psychiatrist from Beth Israel Deaconess Medical Center and assistant professor of psychiatry at Harvard Medical School, recently published an article in the *New England Journal of Medicine* which highlights our patients' desires and expectations to be treated by doctors that are well behaved [2]. As thoughtful practitioners, we are well aware of the humanistic and caring qualities that are required for the most effective healthcare delivery. However, Kahn speculates that many "patients may care less about whether their doctors are reflective and empathic than whether they are respectful and attentive [2]." Dr. Kahn notes

R. Colgan, *Advice to the Young Physician*,
DOI 10.1007/978-1-4419-1034-9_7,
© Springer Science+Business Media, LLC 2009

that most patients complain, not of being misunderstood or denied empathy, but rather of physician behaviors they perceive as rude or neglectful. Dr. Kahn believes that good manners can be learned; moreover, he elucidates how physicians should be reminded to cultivate these behaviors so as to practice "etiquette-based medicine [2]."

Dr. Kahn explains how it is simpler to change physician behavior than patient attitudes:

> Etiquette-based medicine would prioritize behavior over feeling. It would stress practice and mastery over character development. It would put professionalism and patient satisfaction at the center of the clinical encounter and bring back some of the elements of ritual that have always been an important part of the healing professions [2].

Indeed, there exist many behaviors that are not only expected by the patient, but are seen as standards of care by many institutions. Thus, there has evolved many suggestions for physicians providing care to hospitalized patients to act in a way that is valued by patients. The following checklist, also reported in the *New York Times*, offers six simple behaviors that are shown to be perceived by the patient as professional and attentive [3].

The Six Habits of Highly Respectful Physicians

1. Ask permission to enter the room and wait for an answer before doing so.
2. Introduce yourself, showing your ID badge.
3. Shake hands with your patient (wear gloves if needed).
4. Sit down and smile if appropriate.
5. Briefly explain your role on the patient's healthcare team.
6. Ask the patient how he or she is feeling about being in the hospital and listen to the response.

Etiquette-based medicine is such a simple, obvious necessity in the practice of medicine. So much so, that you almost have to wonder why is it being promoted at all. Isn't this already the standard of care? Don't physicians aspire to practice medicine through good behavior? The answers to these questions are not straightforward and are unfortunately compounded by the sad reality that these simple expectations are not always met. Etiquette-based medicine is *not* uniformly practiced today. This lack of civility is not unique to medicine, but an insidious social problem that has escalated over time according to Dr. P.M. Forni, a professor at Johns Hopkins University and co-founder of the Johns Hopkins Civility Project. In Dr. Forni's book *Choosing Civility* he makes the suggestion that "we agree on one principle: that a crucial measure of our success in life is the way we treat one another every day of our lives [4]." Dr. Forni cites 25 behaviors, which the civil person exemplifies. Most of these "rules" are important considerations for all members of society and are applicable to physicians as we strive to become the most effective civil healers possible. Those who wish to improve their healing skills may adapt some of these rules in the care of the patient. The 25 "rules" are included below with examples of how they may relate to patient care.

The Twenty-Five Rules of Considerate Conduct

1. *Pay attention*. This is understood as a variation of Hippocrates urging that we observe all, and of Osler's admonition to use all of our senses when caring for the patient.

2. *Acknowledge others*. Introducing ourselves to others in the room and understanding how they may be familiar with our patient is an example of acknowledging others.

3. *Think the best*. It is easy to assume that a patient requesting narcotics is drug seeking, when in fact the patient likely wants relief from a physical or emotional pain. Our challenge is to begin each encounter with a hopeful attitude and optimistic expectations. We must be careful not to pre-judge patients, even though it is known that some patients may be drug seeking.

4. *Listen*. We have already learned that if you listen to the patient they will tell you the diagnosis, and that much can be inferred from non-verbal communications. I observed a great example of a clinician who showed a keen sense of listening. Recently, in explaining an unpleasant event to a colleague and several third

year medical students, the attending took a long deep breath, followed by a long audible exhalation. In observing this, the astute medical student acknowledged, "Deep sigh," gaining information on the attending's mood, opinions, and emotional state that may have not otherwise been obvious from words alone. I was impressed because she showed astute listening skills—not only to the spoken word but to other sounds around her.

5. *Be inclusive.* Certainly the best way we can be inclusive in the medical profession is by honoring cultural diversity through considerate and thoughtful medical practice. Maintaining awareness that many of those whom we see likely come from a different culture—and thus have different values and beliefs about health, life, and death—is critical in delivering optimal care to all.

6. *Speak kindly.* Beginning your interview with something like, "How may I help?" and ending with a simple, "Is there anything else I can do for you?" denotes kindness.

7. *Do not speak ill.* Healers are at their best when they do not criticize the care rendered by others.

8. *Accept and give praise.* One of the best ways to promote well being in our patients is to go out of our way to find something positive in what they have done to positively affect their health and then compliment them for doing so. Encouraging our patients, and having what the American psychologist Carl Rogers calls "unconditional positive regard" is something we can easily do to improve our patient's healthcare experience.

9. *Respect even a subtle "no."* Of course we must respect our patient's wishes when they do not agree with our recommendations; however, we still have an obligation to give proper informed consent as to what may happen if a patient does not follow our advice. It is our duty to provide the patient with all the information necessary to make an educated decision about his or her health. Even in dire circumstances—such as disregarding advice to visit the emergency department when experiencing anginal chest pain—the patient must understand the consequences. Although difficult, it is our obligation to lay down the facts, especially when disregarding professional medical advice may result in the patient's death; after which, if the answer is still "no," we must respect and honor that person's wishes.

10. *Respect other's opinions.* This works in all directions in every relationship in health care. A primary care provider must value the opinions of a consultant, just as a consultant must value the opinions of his or her primary care colleague. We must value the opinions of our patients, with the hope that they will value ours. Understanding these dynamic relationships and being aware to their implications on healthcare delivery will serve our patients well.

11. *Mind your body.* We cannot take good care of our patients if we do not take good care of ourselves. Often the physician puts his or her health to the wayside to accomplish his or her professional duties. We will explore this further in a later chapter, in a section called Physician Heal Thyself.

12. *Be agreeable.* Even though we may disagree with our patient's decision, we must strive to be agreeable and continue to help them in the most effective way possible in the context of that disagreement. As with the example in number nine, although we may not agree with the decision to forego emergency room care, we can still be agreeable. We can agree to disagree in a civil manner.

13. *Keep it down (and rediscover silence).* Psychiatrists seem to have cornered the market on appreciating the value of silence. This is a skill which, when appropriate, we can emulate. Much can be gained from silence. Often, giving the anxious patient an extended period of time to think before they respond to a question will result in information that may have been missed. Be patient, do not assume, and listen. Allowing our patients their time to tell us what is concerning to them is civility at its best.

14. *Respect other people's time.* "Running late" is at the top of most patients' lists of what frustrates them during visits to their doctor's office. Often this is the reality of healthcare delivery, as unexpected situations arise and simply take longer than expected. However, we can try to prevent dissatisfaction through our actions such as being on time to the office, not over-booking inordinately, and—when all else fails—simply apologizing when we are late. This occurred for me recently as I assumed the role of the patient. I had an appointment with a highly respected and very busy physician and still had not been

called back to the room forty-five minutes after my appointed time. I had another meeting to attend, and so I informed his front desk staff that I needed to reschedule. Although I realized he must have had some urgency arise, I was displeased that I had wasted two hours of my time. I was surprised but pleased to answer a call from this physician at five-thirty that night, apologizing for keeping me waiting. This simple gesture showed class and respect.

15. *Respect other people's space.* It is proper to ask for permission to sit down or start an exam when visiting a hospitalized patient.

16. *Apologize earnestly.* We are going to make mistakes in the course of our job. When we do, it is appropriate and necessary to apologize. Gallagher and colleagues reported on patients' and physicians' attitudes regarding the disclosure of medical errors in a 2003 JAMA article that "physicians should strive to meet patients" desires for an apology and for information on the nature, cause, and prevention of errors [5]."

17. *Assert yourself.* Our duty is to assert ourselves for our patients, especially when doing so will result in more comprehensive care. This is not always easy or glamorous and often is the source of conflict—such as appealing for a previously denied authorization for medical care by an insurance company or going to extra lengths to make sure proper information about your patient reaches a consultant. We should all strive to be the physician that "goes the extra mile" for his or her patients.

18. *Avoid (unnecessary) personal questions.* Our job description entails asking personal questions as part of a true physician–patient interaction. The medical consultation room is sometimes referred to as "the confessional," because it is behind these closed doors in which our patients will tell us things they may never tell anyone else. It is a privilege to be in a position to gather this information; furthermore, to possess such trust and patient confidence. Personal questions are needed to gather pertinent information for patient diagnosis, treatment, and follow-up care. Their personal history often has important medical implications. However, this does not give us license to ask personal questions beyond medical necessity to satisfy our own curiosity. While it may be important to ascertain if a patient is

receiving social security disability income, medical assistance food stamps, or the like, it would likely not be necessary to ask someone who by all appearances is not financially depressed about how much money they make. It is our professional duty to use personal information where appropriate and not overstep our privilege by asking inappropriate or irrelevant questions.

19. *Care for your guests.* It is important to have an office that is accommodating to our elderly and disabled patients; moreover, when extra assistance is provided, it should be done so with respect and thoughtfulness.

20. *Be a considerate guest.* When conducting a home visit, we should schedule our appointment at a time that is amenable to both of us, the care provider *and* the patient. In the course of the home visit, we must be respectful of their environment. For example, ask for permission to sit in a certain chair, use a certain area for the exam, or something as simple as washing your hands on the way out shows great consideration.

21. *Think twice before asking for favors.* The physician–patient relationship represents a complex distribution of power. We are a profession of power—gatekeepers to medical information and health services—and help those who are vulnerable. It can be safely argued that we should not, in the course of our caring for the patient, ask for favors from them.

22. *Refrain from idle complaints.* There is no room in our practice for complaints. Common ones such as "The office has overbooked me again," or "The insurance companies keep wringing me dry," or "I am not paid enough for what I do" are known frustrations associated with providing medical care. However, it does no good to practice with such negative attitudes. We must always realize that as bad as we think things may be for us, they are typically much, much worse for those whom we serve.

23. *Accept and give constructive criticism.* Some of the most valuable lessons we can learn come from our patients, as they offer criticism of our care. We should remember that neither the overly flattering nor the overly critical patient is likely accurate in assessing our overall care. But, we can learn from frank comments from our patients. Likewise, we can and should learn from constructive criticism from our colleagues and teachers.

However, it is important to be objective when doing so and not make personal attacks or take criticism personally. Many young physicians may feel disheartened when they receive criticism, but it is important to realize this is because your mentor believes in you and wants to help you be the best you can be. Not only this, but as a student you will make mistakes and you are expected to learn from them. I have witnessed many examples of constructive or necessary criticism that often leaves the student or resident feeling embarrassed. Some of these include the admonition to refrain from chewing gum while seeing a patient as it denotes an air of casualness to the physician–patient visit. Some are more obvious: Frankly, do not wear a low-lying shirt or one that shows a young females navel. Do not sit at the ambulatory care center desk when work is slow and listen to music via headphones, feet up on a chair as if you are at home. Do not arrive more than 30 minutes late for your patient care session—of course with a valid reason—without calling in advance to give notice. Another very important criticism I have reinforced to many students throughout the years is to say you are going to do something, such as follow through on a test, an outstanding report, a phone call, and not do it. As Dr. Woodward would remind you, "Your word is your bond."

24. *Respect the environment and be gentle to animals.* Schweitzer might use this rule to advocate for reverence for life—all life.

25. *Don't shift responsibility and blame.* When I became the medical director of the Family Medicine department, I took over responsibilities for an academic health center that serves close to 40,000 patients per year. I learned a terrific lesson from the practice manager, called the "Triple 'A' approach." The Triple "A" Approach is useful in dealing with a patient who is angry, because of a perceived wrong inflicted upon them by you or your organization. If appropriate, you can often quickly diffuse a volatile situation by (1) Acknowledging that the person is upset, (2) Accepting responsibility (if and when it is yours to own), and (3) Amending the situation as best you can. The following true story provides an example of not shifting blame and accepting criticism.

I walked into an examination room to see a patient, whom I admitted to our local hospital at 2 a.m. for an acute myocardial infarction and was greeted by his glaring stare. After a few minutes of speaking to him, with his arms folded on his chest and his muscles tense, I said to him, "You look angry." He nodded and said, "Yes, I am." When I asked him why he felt this way he eventually opened up and asked if I remembered examining him in the emergency department. Feeling good about the fact that we diagnosed his acute infarction in time to give him thrombolytic therapy and heparin I said, "Yes, I remember." Then he asked me, "Why did you stick your finger in my behind?" Apparently, unbeknownst to me, my patient was angry that I performed a standard rectal exam (so as to be sure he was not with an occult gastrointestinal bleed that might preclude the safe use of anticoagulation therapy). I realized that I must have done a poor job of explaining why it was necessary to do this exam, and failed to convey how it was standard practice of care that would be conducted for any other patient in his situation. He felt violated. After acknowledging his anger, I accepted responsibility for not explaining to him why this particular exam was important. I then looked to make amends by promising him that I would attempt to be more careful in the future with other patients, should this situation ever arise again. At the end of the visit we were friendly with each again—but I learned a valuable lesson about proper communication from this encounter. More importantly, I accepted responsibility for my patient's dissatisfaction and changed my behavior in future practice to avoid its reoccurrence.

The works of Drs. Kahn and Forni are critical in understanding how best to practice the art of medicine. While it is important to be competent, altruistic, virtuous, well-meaning, and all of the other character traits that constitute a physician successful in practicing the art of medicine, these authors highlight the need to translate good training, intentions, and medical practice into behaviors that are perceived by the patient as being proper, civil, respectful, and professional. One might consider taking an inventory of how you are going to be respectful before you visit your next patient as impractical or obvious, but from my experience, I do not think our patients feel this way. If anything, patients are impressed by such attention to detail regarding their satisfaction of care. Osler might have argued that you are faithfully following two of his cardinal teachings: method and thoroughness. If each of us were competent in practicing etiquette-based medicine and did so at all times, we would not need to be reminded of this. But if we are honest with ourselves, we may admit that there are times when fatigue, inattentiveness and may be just being rushed have led to patient interactions that are less civil than our personal ideals. Be aware of yourself, your patients, and how your behaviors, actions, and mannerisms affect their healthcare experiences.

References

1. *The Genuine Works of Hippocrates: Decorum*. Trans. F. Adams. Philadelphia, PA: Williams and Wilkins, 1939.
2. Kahn, M.. "Etiquette Based Medicine." *N Engl J Med* 2008, 358:1988–1989.
3. Kahn, M.. "The Six Habits of Highly Respectable Physicians." *New York Times*. 3 Dec 2008, late ed. 22 Apr 2009 <http://www.nytimes.com/2008/12 /02/ health/02etiq.html?src=tp>
4. Forni, P. *Choosing Civility: The 25 Rules of Considerate Conduct*. New York: St. Martin's Griffin, 2002.
5. Gallagher, T. and Waterman, A.. "Patients and Physicians' Attitudes Regarding the Disclosure of Medical Errors." *JAMA* 2003, 289: 1001–1007.

Further Reading and Resources

Civility

Small, J., et al., *Improving Your Bedside Manner: A Handbook for Physicians to Develop Therapeutic Conversations with Their Patient*. Austin, TX: Eupsychian Press, 2008.

Cassell, E.J. *The Healers Art*. Cambridge, MA: The MIT Press, 1985.

Moise, H.. *Physician-Patient Relations: A Guide to Improving Satisfaction*. Chicago: IL: American Medical Association Press, 1999.

Ludwig, J. "Physician-Patient Relationship." University of Washington School of Medicine. 11 Apr 2008. Accessed: 30 Apr 2009. <http://depts.washington.edu/ bioethx/topics/physpt.html>.

"Defining the Patient-Physician Relationship for the 21st Century." American Healthways and Johns Hopkins 3rd Annual disease Management Outcomes Summit. Phoenix, AZ. 30 Oct 2003. Accessed: 30 Apr 2009. <http://www.patient-physician.com/docs/PatientPhysician.pdf>

Owens, D. *Hospitality to Strangers: Empathy and the Physician-Patient Relationship*, Atlanta, GA: American Academy of Religion Book, 1999.

Chapter 8
Lessons Learned from Private Practice

Abstract Private practice helps the young physician understand what the standard of care is in your community. Deviation from the standard of care can lead to an allegation of malpractice if harm has been done to the patient. Advice on how to avoid malpractice is given within the context of striving for a higher goal: choosing good practice. Another benefit of private practice is the long-term relationships you develop with your patients. By getting to know your patient better you may best be able to appreciate what Osler described as "the true poetry of life". Stories, sad and humorous, highlighting some of these poetic moments are given as examples from one's private practice.

8.1 Choosing Good Practice

It's smart to avoid malpractice. It's smarter to choose good practice. Good doctors, young and old, practicing good medicine, charting good medical records still get sued. So how can you avoid this? In this section we will give you some tips on how to keep the threat of a lawsuit to a minimum.[1]

---

[1] Originally published in a modified format in *Maryland Family Doctor*, Winter 2009 and authored by Colgan, Richard; Colgan Kathleen, and Farley, Robert.

R. Colgan, *Advice to the Young Physician*,   109
DOI 10.1007/978-1-4419-1034-9_8,
© Springer Science+Business Media, LLC 2009

8.1.1 Definition of Malpractice

Medical malpractice suits fall under the categorization of personal injury or tort law, of which there are three different classifications: negligence, strict liability, and intentional torts. These causes of action are civil (not criminal) and address liability and the nature and extent of damages. Malpractice suits arise when a patient alleges negligence committed by a professional healthcare provider. To prove negligence, a court must find that the healthcare provider deviated from the standard of care deemed reasonable by those with similar training and experience, under similar circumstances, and that this breach in their performance of duties caused harm or injury to a patient. Usually other doctors are called to testify as expert witnesses and give their opinion as to whether a healthcare provider's actions fell below the accepted standard of care and to testify as to what a competent physician would have done under the same or similar circumstances. Thus, the standard for malpractice is set by the medical profession itself, by its own practices and customs.

8.1.2 Common Lawsuits

Before discussing some common malpractice situations, it should be emphasized that the best practices in the physician–patient relationship entail good communication with the patient, and where appropriate (and with the patient's permission) their family. Being sure that your patient understands what you do is critical. At times having that understanding written down and signed is even better. All of us have made mistakes, and most physicians will tell you that with each patient a "credit account" exists whereupon errors or withdrawals are tallied compared with the more common "good doctoring" deposits. The truth is that most patients respect their physicians and few bring malpractice suits. So while it is important that you practice good medicine and document well, the most important reason why a patient does *not* bring a suit against a doctor is their interpretation of a satisfactory physician–patient relationship that has developed, both over time, and especially around the time of the alleged transgression.

Leading the list of common medical malpractice suits are those cases under the heading of undiagnosed or late diagnosis of a catastrophe that ended in either significant morbidity or mortality for the patient. A few common examples of perceived or real errors that led to a claim of medical malpractice follow.

8.1.2.1 Missed Myocardial Ischemia

Failure to appreciate that ischemia can present with epigastric pain, dyspnea, or other atypical symptoms is a common mistake. Similarly is the error of ordering an electrocardiogram, only to erroneously conclude that your patient does not have a myocardial infarction because the electrocardiogram appears normal. The teaching pearl is: If you think that someone may be having acute coronary syndrome based on the history, there are a few particular things on the physical exam or electrocardiogram which may likely mitigate that risk. This is where clinical judgment comes in. The risk of myocardial infarction is higher if there is a gallop, hypotension, pain radiating to both arms; and less if the pain is pleuritic and reproducible by palpating the chest wall.

8.1.2.2 Missed Acute Abdomen

The classical presentation of acute appendicitis is well known, however, patients often present in a non-classical fashion. Two elements in the typical history of appendicitis are the presence of anorexia and the determination that the patient's pain or whatever specific descriptive of "dis–ease" they may use, is constant. One of the best predictors that your patient may be suffering from appendicitis is if the pain is reported (you may have to ask them) to have moved from the periumbilical area to the right lower quadrant. Other subtle findings for non-classical appendicitis are the presence of Dunfy's sign: abdominal pain with coughing; Rovsings sign: right lower quadrant pain with palpation of the left lower quadrant; Iliopsoas test: abdominal pain with extension of the right leg against resistance; and jar tenderness: guarding or pain with sudden movements such as bumping the examining table, jumping in place, or hitting the patient's heel.

8.1.2.3 Failing to Inform Your Patient that They Are a High-Risk Patient

Another general category of malpractice risk is failure to explain to the patient or his or her family just how truly sick the patient is. This is particularly true when you have not yet had the time to develop a longitudinal relationship with your patient. This occurs commonly in instances when you see a new patient that you immediately identify as being very sick or with a high likelihood of an impending catastrophe. In situations like this it may be appropriate to "hang crepe paper," i.e., to explain to the patient and family that your assessment concludes that he or she may be suffering from a very serious condition, and that if this is indeed the true diagnosis it entails a high risk of further morbidity or mortality. Unfortunately such life-threatening illnesses do occur and it is the physician's responsibility to inform the patient that they have, for example, lung cancer, pancreatic cancer, or similar conditions where the life expectancy may be as little as 6 months. Another example is that of a new patient who presents to you with New York Heart Association Class 4 congestive heart failure, which also carries a high risk of death. The term "hanging crepe paper" draws from an old custom of pinning black paper around the home's parlor entrance when death of its inhabitant was perceived imminent.

8.1.3 What Your Defense Attorney Wants You to Know

Just because a patient files a lawsuit against you, does not mean that it possesses legal or factual merit. Therefore, the task for the practitioner is learning how to best avoid becoming a malpractice defendant in the first place; further, if you *are* sued it is important to know what you can do to most effectively assist your defense team (your attorney and malpractice carrier) in representing you.

Many malpractice suits are filed because a patient or his or her family is surprised by the result(s) of a course of treatment or intervention. Often this is because of a perceived incorrect or "missed" diagnosis or is consequence to a family's frustration with a "bad outcome." If patients and their families are able to understand the proposed treatment or intervention in the context of the patient's pre-existing medical condition(s), as well as realize the reality of the less-than-perfect state of medicine—that an outcome cannot be guaranteed or controlled—then there is less "surprise" experienced if something bad happens to the patient. It therefore follows that open and frank discussions with the patient and family are paramount in diminishing the surprise of a bad outcome and hopefully quelling the need for a lawsuit.

By far, the most significant "weapon" in your malpractice defense arsenal is the patient's medical chart and your own proper charting in the records. For a malpractice case to survive preliminary legal challenge, the patient's attorney must secure an independent review of the medical records by another healthcare provider. This person is ultimately required to opine, based on review of the records, that there has or has not been a deviation from applicable standards of care. So, the patient's medical record is both your "sword and shield" as its review might result in the failure of the patient to secure the requisite reviewer's critical opinion and moreover, if suit follows through, the record becomes the foundation of your defense to the alleged negligence. It is imperative that you do your reasonable best to chart clearly, accurately, and timely. However, that does not mean writing a novel for each patient encounter. Rather, note the time of your hospital chart entries as well as when exactly you saw the patient in an effective manner so that a timeline of your patient encounters can be re-created after the fact. Enter a brief summary of discussions you have with the patient, family, and other providers that are of significance to the patient's care (such as passing of orders of a specific nature to a consultant). Write a brief sentence or two of your reasoning for recommending a certain treatment, especially when there may be some disagreement as to its efficacy. Make your charts thorough but concise, keeping in mind that if a suit comes around, the properly documented patient chart is your best defense against any malpractice allegations.

If you are served with a lawsuit, you should first preserve the integrity of the patient's medical record. Insure that the record is in a safe place to begin with (that is, do not "lose or misplace it"). Most importantly, under no circumstances should you endeavor to edit, change, delete, or seek to complete or embellish any of the past entries you or any other individual has made in the patient's medical record! When—not if—discovered, this will result in dire consequences for you and your medical career. If a clinician were to make edits or alterations to the medical record, you should clearly indicate that you are looking to amend the record, reasons for the changes, and the date/time that the changes are made.

Next, you must notify your malpractice insurance carrier of the lawsuit. Remember, even before you have been served with court papers, the patient has already found a lawyer who has investigated the case and deemed it significant enough to follow through with a suit. Therefore, there should be little delay in this notification. You want the carrier to get up to speed as soon as possible in preparing the defense of your case, which includes opening a case file and securing defense counsel on your behalf. Avoid the understandable instinct to speak to others about the fact of this lawsuit or the specifics of your care and treatment of the patient-plaintiff other than representatives of your insurance carrier and your attorney's office. Loose lips sink ships. When speaking to your representatives, speak truthfully, openly, and candidly about the facts of the case and the allegations as you understand them. The defense team will best be able to represent and defend your interests if you tell the truth, even if the truth is "bad, negligent or ugly."

Work with your malpractice carrier and your defense counsel in developing your theory of defense and offering assistance "on the medicine" aspect of the case. This team truly has the successful defense of your interests as their primary objective. Consider engaging in the academic exercise of the reasons that medically and factually your care, management, and treatment met the applicable standards of care and did not cause the patient's alleged injury. By doing so, you will have taken the important first step in developing the defense theory for your case. The defense of a malpractice lawsuit is truly a team effort in which you are a significant contributor! Not only that but you have the most at stake.

Finally, your attorney will keep you advised of the process of the litigation, answer your questions, and counsel you throughout. He or she is your advocate and you should not hesitate to ask him or her questions as to the proposed strategy in defending you, as well as the consequences of any feasible outcome. While medical errors may be inevitable, you can choose to lessen your risk of being served with a malpractice suit. Being aware of the type of clinical scenarios which are more commonly the reason for filing suits, establishing good rapport with your patients, including a frank discussion about their conditions, and contacting your malpractice carrier's legal team as soon as you are concerned about an incident are absolutely critical. The litigation process is dynamic, so maintaining an open line of communication with defense is a must. And, you will survive!

8.2 Searching for the True Poetry of Life

Here's the good news. Almost every one of you, once you are a licensed M.D. or professionally acknowledged healer in service to mankind, will be in the top several percent of wage earners in the world. As highly educated, respected members of your community, you will spend your working days using your training to help others. What a great and fulfilling way to make a living! The down side is that you are entering into a field that requires you to work extremely hard, commit to long hours and rough days, as well as deal with many emotionally stressful situations. There will be times when you wonder if it was all worth it. You will see friends that earn more money than you, perhaps seemingly experiencing fewer difficulties in their occupations. You will have bad days when you simply wonder—why did I get into this field anyway? Osler has a suggestion on how you may stay enthusiastic, when things look dark:

> Nothing will sustain you more potently than the power to recognize in your humdrum routine, as perhaps it may be thought, the true poetry of life—the poetry of the commonplace, of the ordinary man, of the plain, toil-worn woman, with their loves and their joys, their sorrows and their griefs [1].

Searching for the poetry of life is not merely another checkbox to be completed after each patient visit; it does not fall in line right after documenting vital signs and recording the review of systems. Rather, this adage encourages us to be cognizant of the human side of our patients. Or, as one doctor once described to me, "Acknowledge the patient's underside, their soft belly side, the side they do not show the rest of society." One of the many privileges of being a healer is that patients are willing to share this side with us. I am astounded at how often I think I know a patient, only to learn later more about this person's "poetry of life." It also reminds me why I love medicine so much. What follows is the story of one patient whom I met, which exemplifies Osler's quote and truly touched my heart.

He Apologized, Twice

One night while working late at the health center, and in the middle of one of the worst downpours of rain I had ever witnessed, out of the corner of my eye, I caught sight of a man lumbering into our waiting room soaking wet. I judged him to be no more than 30 years old, but what was remarkable about him was that he walked slowly with the aid of two mid-thigh-high wooden walking sticks. This was towards the end of a 12-hour day of seeing patients in our inner city academic primary care clinic—I remember I was longing to go home. I also remember asking myself, "I wonder which doctor is going to see him?" and answering my own question, "I bet it will be me."

At nearly ten 'til seven, the medical assistant asked me if I wanted my 6 PM patient, who had only just arrived, to reschedule. Not knowing it was the same man I had seen earlier, I said, "No, I'll see him." This was how I met Michael.

When I walked into the examining room, I was initially intrigued by Michael's appearance. It was only later that I became aware of his humanity. What was most striking about him was his head of tangled hair. It was neither well combed nor recently washed, and foretold what I might see while looking over the man. When we did make eye contact, I remember thinking how strikingly innocent and needful he was.

Michael's coat was as old and worn as the library book he was reading, the title of which surprised me. In his hand he held an esoteric philosophy textbook that I imagined had not been checked out by anyone for many years. I felt badly for having noticed several old and new stains on his shirt, and was slightly embarrassed to be so obviously better dressed than he was. He did not have control of his body, and he would occasionally twist this way and that. His mouth struggled when he spoke. He had difficulty holding his body still or making it do simple things like laying down his book, which he did when I entered the exam room.

"'I' am sorry I was late," he said before I had the chance to introduce myself. Suddenly, filled with curiosity, I wanted to know more about him. I was surprised to learn, that his parents, whom I used to take care of when I practiced elsewhere years ago, had referred Michael to me. I recalled 5 years earlier that a silver-haired couple sat in a different exam room, in another city miles away, and told me how they were looking forward to moving to a warmer climate in California. They spoke in passing of their only son, Michael, who lived in the city where I now worked and who had been born with a neuromuscular disorder. Although they expressed some concern about moving away, they exhibited calmness about them that I reassured myself had been earned as a reward for decades of successful parenting. They seemed to be confident he would do well. "Would you be his doctor?" they asked, upon learning that I too was leaving to practice in the same city.

Checking Michael's records, I learned that he had sought my help once before, but was seen by another physician in my absence. A year earlier, a potentially life-threatening infection prompted his direct admission to our hospital, after which he underwent emergency surgery. Several months later, he was discharged from a rehabilitation unit to return home and care for himself again. So many questions ran through my head during the first few minutes of our encounter. Did his parents come to see him? Did he have friends to visit him? Did his neighbors watch out for him? Would he be missed at the mailbox if something happened and he didn't show? I was struck then with his seemingly lonely independence.

The purpose of tonight's visit was for a refill of an antidepressant medication. We talked about the book he was reading, and he sought my opinion as to whether or not he would be able to resume a search for employment once again. Throughout the visit I was struck with how different he looked from the man I saw in the waiting room, and how accommodating his behavior was to me, the doctor, the one he needed right now to get a refill for an expensive pill that helped treat his mental illness. How did he afford this medication on a disability income? After finding samples in our drug closet of what he needed, we worked out a plan for a follow up visit. Standing up from the stool (a doctor's cue that the visit is over), I extended my hand and told Michael I looked forward to seeing him again. Still apologetic, he attempted to close the visit by whispering once again, "I'm sorry I was late." Patients have apologized to me before for this very reason, and often I accept their apology and continue my day without giving it a second thought. Sensing there was more he wanted to say I asked, "Why were you late, Michael?" I was not prepared for his answer.

I learned that Michael relies on public transportation. This was the reason he didn't move with his parents, for the bus system where they live is nowhere near as good as in our city. On this night he told me, he had taken the No. 7 bus from his apartment across town to the closest stop near our health center. He walked the remaining twelve blocks from the bus stop, in heavy rain, with the aid of his two wooden walking sticks. I asked how long it had taken him to make this trek down the rainy street, and without expression he replied, "About 20 minutes." I was shocked. This must have been excruciatingly difficult for a person in his physical condition.

At the 1996 Democratic National Convention, Christopher Reeves, the actor who suffered a grave spinal cord injury, gave an unforgettable speech. Some of what he said in his speech reminded me of Michael and his family. I wondered how well I serve patients with disabilities, or patients who came from another culture. As he sat tightly belted in his wheelchair, Mr. Reeves mesmerized his audience, as he said

> Over the last few years we've heard a lot about something called family values. And like many of you I've struggled to figure out what that means. But since my accident I've found a definition that seems to make sense. I think it means we're all family, and that we all have values. And if that is true, if America really is family, then we have to recognize that much of our family is hurting [2].

These thoughts filled my mind as I looked at Michael. If Michael was hurting that night he didn't complain to me, his physician. How could he not have been hurting after such a difficult struggle to get here? The image of this civil, soft-spoken, disabled man is perhaps familiar to many of us. He may have been like many men we see on a city street corner, an image that cues us to turn the other way. If our eyes meet we are forced to face something that is painful and easier to ignore.

The fact that a member of our family felt the need to apologize *twice* for the slight inconvenience he had caused me, while on this search for self-betterment, has to touch your heart; that Michael's story represents but one of many more which go unnoticed should make us weep. As medical practitioners, we have been given a special opportunity, a privilege, to share in an intimate and helpful relationship with patients from our culture, as well as, those from completely different backgrounds. In our fast-paced practices, it is easy to get consumed by busy days and tight schedules. Further, the increasing dominance of technology in medical practice creates an atmosphere that makes it easy to trivialize the need and value of the healer's art.

What can we—as healers—take away from Michael's story? One lesson may be that while we are here to serve mankind, we do so one person at a time, and those whom we serve are in need of our care. Perhaps we need to remind ourselves to listen more actively so that we may hear our patients, and cue into what makes them unique and special individuals. If we do not look outside our culture, we may miss meeting other members of our human family. Most importantly, if we overlook the opportunity to extend our hand to someone in need, we will ultimately be the ones that find ourselves alone and unfulfilled.

Michael never returned to see me for his follow-up visit. Two years after I initially encountered him, I came across Michael waiting in another exam room on another doctor's schedule. I asked if it would be alright if I saw him, and he said yes. He told me that since we last met he had been diagnosed with a more serious mental illness and was hospitalized for several months. He was still looking for a job, and still loved to read. I did my best to reconnect with Michael, and urged him to come back and see me, so that I may be his regular doctor. He said he would. From this experience with Michael, I have changed my practice for the better. Now, if a patient arrives late, I think twice about asking him or her to reschedule and try to consider each individual's story. When he didn't keep his follow-up visit, I called Michael's home repeatedly. There was never an answer, and I continue to be unable to reach him. It has been 7 years.

The above story may rightfully be viewed as sad, and to me it is very heart wrenching. My voice deepens every time I tell this story to my students, and I often think of the lessons that can be learned from patients like Michael. Although many situations in medicine are often difficult, some of the most poetic moments we encounter in practice are incredibly positive, uplifting, or just plain funny. I encourage every young healer to keep a log or journal of their more memorable poetic moments from practice. Reading these stories years later, as your wisdom increases and you beliefs evolve will sustain you. What follows are a few entries from a journal I started years ago, when I first began private practice.

8.3 A Doctor's Journal

Osler once explained how "nothing will sustain you more potently than the power to recognize. . .the true poetry of life [1]." I add that it is even better to write it down. As a young physician you are in a great position to begin keeping a diary, journal, or blog in which memorable stories are saved, for you have so many years of experiences ahead of you. I urge you to write down some of these more memorable "doctor stories" and look back on them often.

The American poet and general practitioner William Carlos Williams, (1883–1963) "worked harder at being a writer than he did at being a physician," wrote the biographer Linda Wagner-Martin. Williams felt that being a practitioner of medicine helped him become a better writer. I admit to being inspired by William's *Doctor Stories*, a wonderful collection of tales that I highly recommend to you as further reading, for it illustrates what one practitioner can create by simply putting his or her own stories down on paper. You shouldn't worry that you may not see yourself as the same caliber of writer as Williams. That's not the point. Rather, each one of us has at least one story, which could be published if crafted properly. Below are a few entries from a journal I started in my first year of private practice.

*****

Gregory B. is an adorable 3-year-old boy whose mother brought him in to see me for a number of complaints. He's been suffering from a cough along with some nasal discharge, a bellyache, and some assorted bodily pains, among many other issues. As his mother listed concern after concern, I directed the interview to the preschooler himself. I asked Gregory, "What bothers you the most?" His eyes opened wide as he immediately brought the answer to mind. "Fire...and snakes in the mud!" he chirped. His mother explained that in fact last night he had experienced a nightmare with images of the above; and to that extent she felt this response was accurate.

*****

A smartly dressed, well-spoken gentleman saw me at the office with the chief complaint of sore throat. From the start of the visit, it was clear that he wanted to provide me a very specific and detailed description of his condition. During the course of the interview, the glib man pointed to the normal "punching bag structure" found dangling from posterior aspect of his soft palate (known medically as the uvula). He cited that what bothered him most was his, "Vulva." I immediately asked him to repeat his answer, as I was not sure I heard him correctly. "I saw that my vulva was swollen," he said. I now faced a dilemma: Should I correct him on the proper use of the word "uvula?" Should I ruin this humor for all doctors down the road who might otherwise hear his mistake? I won't tell you my decision.

*****

Children definitely describe symptoms differently than adults. Stephanie B. is a 7-year-old who was experiencing some gastrointestinal distress. She described this innocently as, "It feels like a feather in my throat ... like birds taking a bath in my stomach."

*****

This is another 6-year-old boy, whom I met sitting on the examining table looking annoyed. He had a different chief complaint than what was described in the nurse's note. I asked the boy what bothered him the most, rather than the reported "cough." He looked once towards his parents who were sitting to his left and said, "When I am trying to talk and people, like these two here, interrupt me." When I asked him if anything else bothered him, he said, "Yeah, when I am trying to watch TV and people stand in front of it."

*****

Margaret R. is a 68-year-old proper lady from London, England. I have taken care of her for many years, and over this time we have enjoyed many laughs together. During a routine sigmoidoscopic exam, I asked her if she would like to have a look inside, as I have asked all of my other patients in the past when performing this exam. I explained that if she so chose, this would be accomplished by turning the scope so she, too, could look through the eyepiece. She replied, "That would be quite lovely". As she peered through the scope this cheerful British woman exclaimed, "This is quite marvelous!" After which she questioned, "It rather looks like the planets doesn't it?" To which I replied, "I have never thought of it that way before, but if you had to think of any one planet that it looks like, you'd have to say it looks like Uranus." The nurse bumped into the surgical tray, instruments fell to the floor, and I began to think that perhaps I had gone too far in being familiar and attempts to joke around with my patient. Thoughts of calls to the Board of Physicians by my patient or the surgical nurse began to illogically enter my mind. I didn't see this patient again for a year, and this hiatus convinced me that indeed I had offended her and prompted her to seek care elsewhere. When she did return a year later I greeted her with a warm, "Hello," and shortly thereafter told her that I thought she had fired me because of the comment I made during our last visit. "What, no, I am sorry," she said, "I don't remember that." As it turned out she moved back to England to care for a sick relative and had not given the off-colored joke a second thought. She and I were both happy to continue our special physician–patient relationship.

****

I hope reading these entries will encourage you to begin your own collection of writings. As memorable events occur, you will discover that they grow dim over time and are eventually forgotten. Surely, looking back on what you considered to be significant experiences throughout the years will bring you back—not only to those events themselves—but to that time and place, to the life events surrounding you then. These memories are true treasures. They perk you up after depressing or difficult days. They ground you when you feel overwhelmed. They remind you why you became a healer, and hopefully inspire you to continue your extraordinary work.

8.4 Physician Heal Thyself

You cannot reach your full potential as a healer, if you do not look after yourself—your physical, social, and emotional well-being. Many physicians I know seem to wear their lack of routine health care as a badge of honor. As if to take time out and have another physician help you with your own health is in some way selfish. It is quite the contrary; it is foolish. The practice of medicine is demanding, and the toll it can take on a physician is significant and not to be neglected. Dr. Theodore Woodward notes in his book, *A Time for Sentiment*, that "the likelihood for suicide, like addiction, is high in physicians." He explains how "this is perhaps understandable when one considers the intense need to acquire knowledge, the drive to excel, and the intense worry about decision making and its consequences." Unfortunately too many physicians, and perhaps their families, go without the same good medical care they diligently recommend and provide to their patients. While fewer physicians smoke cigarettes today than in previous years, many do not follow through on important preventive medicine strategies, such as colonoscopy, hypertension screening, or other important medically recommended procedures. We must also look out for our personal well-being, in the same way we should get a flu shot each year. Missing work because of a preventable illness or compromising your ability to deliver care because of disregard for your own health only denies your patients proper access to health care.

I have known doctors (including a gastroenterologist) who were diagnosed with advanced colon cancers, due to lack of proper colorectal cancer screening. I know physicians who care for adult patients, but do not know their own blood pressure or cholesterol level. When you care for yourself or loved ones, it becomes difficult to draw the line and even easier to overstep those drawn by professional medical societies and ethics committees. When you or a loved one is sick, seek out another physician for treatment.

One summer, I served as an "able-bodied" seaman for the Association of Maryland Pilots. One night near Norfolk, Virginia, I assisted a Chesapeake Bay pilot to the ship's ladder at 2 AM, amidst gale-force winds raging up the Chesapeake Bay. As the 30-foot launch heaved up and down alongside this inbound container ship, I had difficulty tying the bag to the rope needed to carry it topside. We both were in danger of going overboard. The senior pilot urged me to look out for myself while performing the dangerous tasks required by this job. He yelled to me through the wind, "One hand for yourself and one hand for the ship." This maritime adage applies to us in medicine as well. Healers should not feel guilty about looking after themselves, even if doing so comes before delivery of care to their patients. By being healthy ourselves, we may live another day to take good care of our patients and moreover to make sure the care we provide is the most effective and successful possible. My advice to this end is that every healer should find someone they have confidence in and seek their care. Be it preventive or treatment, you have the right to receive expert care. Not only this, but your patients deserve to have you at the peak of wellness, so that you can best serve them. Too often physicians—being physicians in conveniently close proximity to medical care—will self-diagnose and treat themselves. Even worse, they extend this care to their family. Although most of us do this to some extent, it starts us down the path to crossing those lines. In treating our loved ones, we are unable to be objective and less likely to be as thorough. The care we provide to them is skewed by our connection, and often it is substandard to care provided by someone else. The best way a physician can heal himself is to seek the advice of a trusted healer, and follow it.

Another important way to look after yourself is to realize that in any service industry, including health care, we may find ourselves in threatening situations. Fortunately this is rare in most fields of medicine, but as a public servant we may sometimes be confronted with people who look to harm us. The following two true stories illustrate this point. Some patients are overly friendly, because that is their nature, or the way in which they want to express appreciation. Other patients are overly friendly, or look to attach themselves to their healers because of frank mental illness. I admire the intent of physicians who give out their home and cell phone numbers or provide their home addresses so that patients may easily contact them. I admit to doing this rarely, because I have seen first-hand what mental illness can do to a patient, in distorting his or her interpretations of reality and social boundaries. I was stalked by one of my patients, and I wouldn't wish this experience on anyone. What follows is an account of this interaction, which I am anxious to tell you about for one reason only: I hope you never have to go through what I went through.

For privacy reasons, I will go out of my way to not be specific in the details of this interaction. Suffice it to say that I saw a patient in my private practice years ago for a rather straightforward complaint and recommended an appropriate, standard of care, evaluation and management plan. This was followed by several back and forth increasingly bizarre interactions with this patient, which caused me to be concerned. I couldn't understand why I was receiving single-spaced, multiple-paged letters by this patient alleging mistreatment and malpractice. I was threatened with being reported to multiple oversight agencies for my bad doctoring. I felt then, as I know now, that I had done nothing wrong. I had the foresight to discharge the patient from my practice in proper legal format, i.e., in writing, with 30 days notice and offering to forward medical records to another physician upon receipt of a written directive to do so. Nonetheless, the patient continued to stalk me by phone, mail, and in person, informing me that the discharge was not accepted until I righted the perceived wrong that I had done. I began to fear for my family's safety, as I thought this person was truly out of their mind. This nightmare got worse. I was reported to the State Board of Physicians, a federal office that dealt with the rights of those with disabilities and our states' medical assistance office. I sought the counsel of an attorney. I told him my story, and he reached into his bookshelf pulling down a state law text. The attorney opened to a page describing in detail what was happening to me; it was the state law on harassment.

I was advised that I could go before a judge and get a restraining order. I reflected upon what I had learned in behavioral pediatrics, as I thought this person's behaviors were childlike and represented a type of acting out at a minimum. I did not know then with certainty that the person was certifiably mentally ill. I remembered that if you want to extinguish a certain behavior in a child, it is better to not attend to the behavior, but rather to ignore it. I decided against pursuing the restraining order, as I thought it might add fuel to the fire. Two months later this patient was admitted for their first paranoid schizophrenic break, which was later followed by many more psychiatric hospitalizations. In retrospect, my patient's abnormal pursuit of me represented the early signs of psychiatric illness. This taught me an important lesson: Physician – protect yourself.

Protecting yourself is not self-centered, but represents good medical practice. The example above is of course extreme, but there are many ways to avoid or abate dangerous situations should they arise. Examples include sitting near an open door when you perceive a patient to be hostile, making sure to have an attendant present—of the opposite sex—when performing sensitive parts of the physical exam (e.g., the pelvic or genital exam). Additionally, you want to be careful when examining an acutely psychotic paranoid schizophrenic patient. Be careful not to be perceived as threatening, and if need be simply stop the exam and walk away. I declined to examine a patient like this when requested to perform the admission exam at a local psychiatric hospital, diffusing the situation to avoid the possibility of physician harm. Instead I spoke with him in the hallway, where I could exit easily. During the exam, I was struck by how paranoid he appeared. After asking him if I may listen to his back, I noticed his spine straightened and he became very rigid. Something told me that I should be frightened of this unfortunate patient. I concluded the exam and thanked him for his time. The next day I was asked to attend to the same psychiatric hospital's staff psychiatrist, who suffered a stab to the neck from the very same patient. She had come physically too close to this patient and was unable to protect herself when he snapped. I believe there is no greater satisfaction than to serve, but the wise healer recognizes that he or she must be in good physical condition in order to serve well and is aware that there will be rare instances when you must be mindful of your own personal safety.

References

1. Osler, W.. "The Student Life." *Aequanimitas: With Other Addresses to Medical Students, Nurses and Practitioners of Medicine*. Philadelphia, PA: P. Blackiston's Son and Co., 1907. 404–405.
2. Reeve, C.. The Christopher Reeve Homepage, "We, The People", <http://www.chrisreevehomepage.com/editorial-wethepeople.html>, accessed May, 2009.

Further Reading and Resources

Searching for the True Poetry of Life

Colgan, R. "I am Sorry I was Late." *Acad Med* 2002, 77(10): 946.

Williams, W. *The Doctor Stories*. New York: New Directions Publishing Corporation, 1984.

A Doctors Journal

Taylor, R.B. *The Clinician's Guide to Medical Writing*. New York: Springer, 2005

Physician Heal Thyself

Angres, D., et. al. *Healing the Healer: The Addicted Physician*. Maddison, CT: Psychosocial Press, 2001.

Chapter 9
The Healer

Abstract What does the consummate healer look like? How can he or she be recognized from among the many technicians who practice the healing arts? Characteristics of the ideal healer are reviewed and categorized into three areas: The physician's individual characteristics as a person; the nature of the physician–patient relationship; and the physician and how he defines his role in society, particularly one who looks to serve more than an individual patient, but humankind.

Je le pansais, Dieu le guérit.

I bandaged them, God healed them.
— Ambrose Paré [1]

How does the consummate, flawless healer come to manifest? We do not and cannot know, because he or she does not exist. Just as we cannot define what perfection or pure beauty is, we must reconcile that such a declaration is not a fact, but an opinion. Throughout the ages, many great teachers of the *art* of medicine have both spoken about and lived exemplary lives that demonstrate what most of us— from both the medical and lay communities—would likely agree is the essence of the consummate healer. While it may be difficult to define the art of medicine, most people can often tell you that they know it when they see it. But where is this notion written?

The young physician who strives to make the transition from technician to healer deserves to be educated as to what makes

R. Colgan, *Advice to the Young Physician*,
DOI 10.1007/978-1-4419-1034-9_9,
© Springer Science+Business Media, LLC 2009

a great healer. He or she must take on this journey to improve their own abilities and, if for no other reason, to know what gold standard to aspire to. Even if perfection is not obtainable in the pursuit of the ideal physician–patient relationship, we owe it to our patients to attempt to define this concept as it embodies the art of medicine. Moreover, once this bar is made visible, we have a duty to try to achieve such a level of care even if we fail. We must strive for perfection and complete ideals for the betterment of our patients.

The young healer might reasonably ask, "Who do I turn to for advice?" I suggest that we begin by identifying role models known to each of us, whether we be a student, young physician, or more seasoned clinician. These are the "ordinary" physicians in our community who on a daily basis are doing the extraordinary by virtue of how they practice medicine, in an exceptional manner with little formal recognition or fame. However, it would be foolish to overlook the collective wisdom, teachings, and examples of those who have gone before us and who have been recognized as distinguished and honored leaders by virtue of how they practiced clinical medicine. No one person can accurately scan the history of medicine and create a list of "best practices" that all physicians would agree to. Despite this, I do not think we should abandon such a quest, as quixotic as it may sound. Then again, maybe like Don Quixote I am delusional. Or perhaps, medical greats such as Osler had this in mind in urging medical students to read Don Quixote, the fictional character of Spanish author Miquel de Cervantes Saavedra (1547–1616). The hero of this epic novel acted upon erroneous fixed beliefs that seemed unreal and unachievable to those around him, while proclaiming proudly:

It is the mission of each true knight. . .

His duty. . . nay, his privilege!

To dream the impossible dream,

To fight the unbeatable foe,

To bear with unbearable sorrow

To run where the brave dare not go;

To right the unrightable wrong [2].

To anyone who believes that the absolutes of patient care are not captured in such poetic advice, I whole-heartedly agree with you. I urge that others attempt to reframe how to best teach today's young physicians on how to be superb clinicians and moreover, that these lessons do not remain vague and are made applicable to common situations encountered in practice. This is not to say I do not appreciate the connection between these poetic teachings and modern medical practice. However, I think that the essence of what we want in a healer is at least suggested below. I offer this book as one physician's effort to carry forth this important and humanistic dialogue, which began centuries ago. By looking to the thoughts, writings, and histories of Hippocrates, Aristotle, Plato, in the Ancient era; to Rhazes, Avicenna, and Maimonides in Medieval times; Osler, Schweitzer, and Peabody in the twentieth century to some of today's modern masters including Pellegrino, Farmer, and Woodward so that we may come to better understand how to practice the art of medicine.

But before we can effectively teach the art of medicine we must identify what it is. In medicine, physicians are not the sole interpreters of what constitutes the ideal physician–patient relationship. The non-medical community has and should always weigh in on what they value in their doctor, for it is those patients who we largely serve. Once we better understand what values and behaviors are cherished by our patients, we can teach these lessons to the young technician who strives to be a true healer.

...To love, pure and chaste, from afar,

To try, when your arms are too weary,

To reach the unreachable star! [2]

Throughout time, cultures have and continue to value the good health of their people. As healers, we are in a fortunate position to improve health and well-being of those we care for. Because of this, we are treated differently—in fact better—rewarded for our hard work and social efforts, recognized for attempting to better humankind. These rewards come in both tangible and intangible forms. Most healers need never be concerned about a mortgage or a car payment. We can typically go out to dinner without worrying about the cost. But as noted by the Apostle Luke, "Much will be required from everyone to whom much has been given. But even more will be demanded from the one to whom much has been entrusted" [3].

The true healer understands that medicine is not just a job but a call to service, a call to help their fellow man, a vocation. It has been said that some doctors suffer from a "God complex," arrogantly thinking themselves above or better than their patients. The role of the physician naturally sets up a disparity in power and knowledge between those giving and receiving care. Unfortunately this power is sometimes abused. We must strive to be humble and grateful for our position in society. Hippocrates sets this record straight, noting in Decorum "The gods are the real physicians" [4]. Likewise we are reminded by the French surgeon Ambrose Pare (1510–1590) that our abilities as physicians are limited—that God heals and we supply the bandages [1]. However, it is not as simple as this. We must still learn how to apply the bandages, to practice the science and art of medicine with a goal of perfection, in recognition of this God-given privilege.

The greatest medical philosophers and teachers of all time are in agreement on several tenets, characteristics of the ideal healer, which can be clearly defined, thanks to either their writings or exemplified by their convictions and the principles by which they lived. In researching the lives and behaviors of some of the most influential physicians through the ages several themes recur throughout the eras. The essential attributes of the healer can be viewed in terms of (1) the character of the individual healer; (2) the behaviors which are seen in the delivery of health care; and (3) how this physician chooses to help others above and beyond the individual physician–patient encounter. In an effort to better communicate these teachings, I list below what I suggest constitutes some of the essential attributes found in the ideal practitioner, one who is recognized by his patients as a master of the Healing Arts—as the perfect healer.

...This is my Quest to follow that star,

No matter how hopeless, no matter how far,

To fight for the right

Without question or pause,

To be willing to march into hell

For a heavenly cause! [2]

9.1 The Healer as a Person

The physician who has mastered the art of medicine has a true interest in humanity and believes there is no higher calling in life than service to his fellow man. He or she is a moral agent, who practices medicine based upon a conviction of pursuing altruistic beneficence. This healer is one who shows respect not only to his or her patients but to family, acquaintances, and self. He or she is described by others as some who is above all civil, polite, and kind in interaction with all contacts, regardless of their station in life. He or she is able to detach from the allure of worldly pleasures so as to be the best healer possible, while remaining humble and knowing the limitations of this exceptional art. I recently asked a group of medical students to describe a healer's personal attributes. They described him or her as someone who was empathetic, selfless, giving, and personable. This healer is depicted as hard working, a constant learner who is respectful, approachable, thoughtful, compassionate, honest, and caring. Other noted qualities included kindness, being nonjudgmental, wisdom, realistic as well as idealistic, understanding, patient, curious, and someone who is able to maintain a broad perspective and an open mind.

> ...And I know, if I'll only be true
>
> To this glorious Quest,
>
> That my heart will lie peaceful and calm
>
> When I'm laid to my rest [2].

9.2 The Healer–Patient Interaction

A healer can be seen by others as someone who truly cares for the patient, as he or she always keeps focus on the patient, especially when not under the observation of others. This person understands that if it is not possible to provide help to someone, then at a minimum he or she should "first do no harm." The healer goes out of his or her way to learn from all patients and others who aid in their care. He or she is observant, thorough, methodical, contemplative, and careful. The healer is an independent thinker who practices evidence-based medicine. Nor only this, but he or she does so in the context of providing the most appropriate and effective care possible.

Under stressful situations, the healer exhibits both an inner and outer calmness in the discharge of duties. He or she is not easily flustered or perturbed. All matters between physician and patient are kept confidential, and trust is preserved at all times throughout the duration of the healer–patient relationship. The healer looks to educate patients as to what he or she understands may be beneficial in improving their health, while maintaining openness to learn from them. The consummate healer recognizes that he or she is caring for someone with a disease, a person who is experiencing an illness that affects both them and their family, and not just taking care of a pathological disease process. The healer is temperate and modest in making recommendations. When it comes to therapeutics, he or she is assistive to nature and when felt to be beneficial, looks to incorporate proper diet, exercise, and the patient's activities in the overall care of the patient. Above all else, the healer strives for excellence in every physician–patient relationship.

When I asked the same group of medical students to describe what they would expect to see in the interactions between a healer and his or her patient, they imagined a healer that is skilled in listening to his or her patients and who avoids interruption. This ideal healer is empathetic, is respectful, maintains excellent rapport, and demonstrates a good and wholesome sense of humor. Other attributes they expect of this healing relationship are displayed as the physician ensures patient comfort and allows for two-way communication that establishes a sense of equality between the physician and patient. Moreover, that this relationship is used in an effective way to not only address the patient's health concerns, but to assure that their emotional needs are also being addressed. This ideal healer helps channel a patient's fears and frustrations into hope and action, and accomplishes this while being honest, trustful, and showing a genuine interest in the patient as a person.

9.3 The Healer's Vocation

Someone who has made the transition from technician to healer looks beyond his or her own needs. This individual desires and also recognizes that there is more to medicine than the finite number of individual patients seen throughout his or her lifetime. While each patient is of utmost importance, an exemplary healer is one who also views the betterment of humankind as a personal responsibility. Where inequality in health care exists, the healer accepts the challenge to do what is possible to help society as a whole, particularly those who represent the most vulnerable and disadvantaged populations. The healer acknowledges a personal accountability for his or her actions, not only to the patients that he or she directly serves but also to their entire community. The healer provides care for the poor and advocates for those who are victimized by healthcare disparities. This is accomplished by diligent observation of patterns of disease amongst the patient population and aim to educate both current and future doctors. Furthermore, the ideal healer is described as one who inspires enduring leadership, volunteers in his or her community, and is a pacifist and an environmentalist. He or she works past social prejudices and provides equal care to all patients, regardless of race, ethnicity, or social background. This person demonstrates love for others by a commitment to service. As an ideal healer, he or she shows respect and honor to the teachers and mentors in the practice of the art and science of medicine.

I encourage the young physician to embrace the science of medicine and to stay current with the highly evolving evidence-based practice of medicine. If we never forget to focus on the quality of care we render to each of our patients, we will likely practice the art of medicine to the best of our abilities. Above all else, the healer is cognizant that their vocation is a sacred and honorable one. We are privileged to watch over our fellow man, to use the lessons bestowed by those who came before us to provide every member of our human family with thoughtful and compassionate medical care.

> ...And the world will be better for this,
>
> That one man, scorned and covered with scars,
>
> Still strove, with his last ounce of courage,
>
> To reach the unreachable stars! [2]

In closing, I offer the following healer's prayer to support each one of us along the way:

A Healer's Prayer

God, let me begin each clinical encounter by always putting my patient's needs first. Grant me the strength to not be seduced by the allure of worldly pleasures, so as to be the best healer I can be, as I look to be thorough and careful in practicing my art.

Guide me as I practice this sacred vocation. May I have the wisdom to learn from the lessons of my teachers, as I contemplate how to best serve each person who seeks my counsel. Help me to use all of my senses as I strive for excellence in caring for my patients, and to understand that if I cannot help someone, then at a minimum I will do no harm. Strengthen me to have an inner and outer calmness when faced with the inevitable difficulties that lie before me.

Show me how to best educate my patients on how to live longer and healthier lives, while being open to learning from those whom I serve. Show me how to be temperate and modest as I look to assist nature by incorporating proper diet, exercise and my patient's own resources in their overall care. Never let me forget that I am caring for someone who is suffering from a disease, and not taking care of a disease. May I never forget my duty to practice medicine based upon a conviction of pursuing altruistic beneficence, marked by showing compassion for others as I commit myself to a life of service.

May I not abandon, but look to serve the poor and advocate for those who suffer because of disparities in our health care system. Remind me to keep matters between physician and patient confidential and that I am accountable for my actions. May I always show respect and care for myself and my family, while being kind in my everyday interactions with others.

I ask you for humility in knowing the limitations of my art. May I always end each encounter with my patient knowing that I have done my best in assisting you by applying the bandages, while taking comfort in the fact that only power greater than I heals.

References

1. *The Apologie and Treatise of Ambroise Pare Containing the Voyages Made Into Divers, with Many of His Writings Upon Surgery*. Ed. Keynes, G. Chicago, IL: University of Chicago Press, 1952.
2. De Cervantes, M. *Don Quijote*. Ed. de Armas Wilson, D. Trans. Burton Raffel. Norton Critical 2nd Ed. New York: W.W. Norton and Co., 1999.
3. Luke, http://bible.cc/luke/12-48.htm, accessed September 9, 2009.
4. *The Genuine Works of Hippocrates*. Trans. F. Adams. Cambridge: Williams & Wilkins Co., 1939.

Further Reading and Resources

Sulmasy, D. *The Healers Calling: A Spirituality for Physicians and Other Health Care Professionals*. Mahwah, NJ: Paulist Press, 1997.
The Institute for the Study of Health and Illness: <http://www.commonweal.org/ishi/>

Index

R. Colgan, *Advice to the Young Physician,*
DOI 10.1007/978-1-4419-1034-9,
© Springer Science+Business Media, LLC 2009